# How to Overcome a Stroke

Mathew Appleton

Strokes happen because the blood flow to part of the brain is disturbed. The effects can be serious or minor, the long term, emotional and physical. If you have a stroke, the more you and the people who care for you understand about the problems it causes the better your chances of leading a normal life again.

If you've been told your at risk of a stroke and need to know the warning signs, or you've had a stroke and want to know how it will affect your life, this is the book for you. If you're caring for someone who's had a stroke and want to help him or her recover, you need this book.

This book will change your attitude to a more optimistic view after a couple of hours browsing. Its store of commons sense, ideas tips and useful information makes it a bargain.... Written with compassion...

# Contents

e

# Introduction

The thought of having a stroke is terrifying. Ask anyone the medical disaster they fear most, and it is odds on that the answer will not be a heart attack, or even cancer.

It's the thought that we might be 'locked in' by a stroke to a paralyzed body, unable to move, touch, feel, talk and generally communicate. To have lost so much in our quality of life and be so totally dependent scares us much more than death itself.

This book is about strokes. It explains why we have them, how we can prevent them, and how we can cope with them. Despite the subject, it's not depressing. For we have come a long way in our understanding of strokes, and in particular, in how we can help stroke sufferers to return towards a normal life.

Even better, we now know how to spot probable stroke victims in time, and how to help them to avoid catastrophe. For although the word 'stroke' suggests an event coming out of the blue, without warning, this is hardly ever the case. Almost every stroke victim has had some warning sign that should have rung the alarm bells. In many of these cases, heeding the alarm in time can help prevent the stroke itself.

So the book is written for three separate audiences. First, for everyone - because the risk of stroke exists in all of us and the way we live can either reduce it, or make it worse. Stroke is one of the diseases of civilization that is thankfully decreasing with better health education and better living conditions.

Second, for carers of stroke victims - who need to know how to bring the best out of them. The story of the actress Patricia Neal, described in Valerie Eaton Griffith's book, A Stroke in the Family, is a shining example of how untrained, but determined and loving, helpers can do so much for a person devastated by a series of severe strokes.

Finally, and most important, for stroke victims themselves. A layman's image of the average stroke victim is of sudden, complete loss of movement, sensation and understanding, perhaps in coma or in a stupefied, hopeless state.

The true picture is usually very different. Most people recover from their stroke with intellect intact. There may be difficulties in talking, in moving about and in vision, but they can all be overcome, at least to some extent, and often totally so. Their greatest problems are the frustration that stroke brings. There is a feeling of helplessness, of loss of control, of being a diminished human being, that must be overcome.

Many stroke victims will be able either to read this book themselves or to appreciate it being read to them. There is nothing in these pages that needs to be hidden from you, or to hinder your optimism about your recovery.

There are times when you will despair of any further recovery, but never give up. Most general practitioners have seen improvements in stroke victims that started months after their attack, and there are always ways to improve the function of the muscles and senses that remain, so that they compensate for those that have been lost.

For the small number of stroke victims who live alone, I make a special plea. Please make sure that you are getting all the help you can from the services around you. Don't try to soldier on alone. Do take advantage of all the people, in the local authority services, and in organizations like Age Concern and The Stroke Association. They will make life so much easier, without invading your privacy.

*Important note*

Throughout the book I generally refer to stroke victims as 'he' and to their carers as 'she'. This is simply for convenience. It cannot be emphasized too strongly that strokes affect both sexes, virtually in equal numbers, and that sufferers are cared for by both men and women.

# 1 Why We Have Strokes

Strokes have the reputation of 'hitting out of the blue'. People are suddenly struck down by them - hence the name. In fact, it's rarely exactly like that.

Before many strokes, there are periods, sometimes only hours long, sometimes lasting for months, in which subtle changes in health warn of impending disaster. Brief moments of blacked out vision, of feelings of weakness in a limb, or loss of sensation; perhaps a persistent early morning headache; a few seconds of unexplained clumsiness, or of inability to think straight.

All these may have other explanations: but they can be signs that the circulation to a part of the brain is under stress, and that it may eventually be shut off completely. When that happens, the stroke begins.

Strokes take several forms. They may cause sudden loss of consciousness, without warning. They may be preceded by headache, weakness and numbness in a limb, a period of confusion, or of disturbances in sensation, such as an odd taste, or smell, or of noises in the head.

The symptoms can progress very quickly to unconsciousness, or slowly increase over hours, so that patients can describe what is happening to them before they eventually 'pass out'.

First aid in stroke cases is basic, but can save lives. There are three essentials:

• Get help as quickly as possible - phone for an emergency ambulance.
• Keep the patient at complete rest and in quiet and peaceful surroundings, with a feeling of competence and reassurance around him.
• Deal properly with unconsciousness.

An unconscious person should be placed on one side, the upper knee drawn up, the head resting on a cushion or pillow so that it is not bent to one side or down on the chin, and so that the breathing is not blocked in any way. Make sure that the tongue is not folded back into the throat, and that false teeth have been removed.

Many stroke victims arrive in hospital with very little information about their immediate past. The hospital staff need to know from whoever has accompanied the patient the circumstances that led up to the stroke, and the immediate past medical history, including all the medicines that he or she has been taking. So any medicines at home must be brought in, so that they can be checked by the hospital staff.

Like its onset, the aftermath of stroke varies, from complete recovery of all sensation and movement, to severe disability. Some stroke victims may be left with no noticeable disability, others, sadly, never recover consciousness. Most recover to a state somewhere between the two, with some weakness and loss of feeling, A few are left with speech difficulties and difficulties in communicating with others. This book is for all stroke victims, no matter how severely afflicted, and for their carers.

*Why strokes happen*

Strokes happen because the blood flow to a part of the brain is disturbed. Within a few minutes the center of that area of brain is damaged, some of it beyond repair. But there is a zone around the most severely affected part - doctors call it the penumbra - that is only partly affected, and, given the correct treatment, will recover. The aim of every stroke treatment is to minimize the area of permanent damage, to maximize the 'rescue' of the penumbra and then to do as much as possible to retrain the healthy part of the brain to take over the job of the lost tissues.

That is this whole book in a nutshell! How we try to accomplish these aims fills the rest of these pages.

First of all, however, it is best to understand something of why stroke occur, and of what is happening in the brain before, during and after a stroke. Once we know that, we can plan the management of the healing period not just more sensibly, but with more sensitivity.

The brain is fed with blood from the heart by three main arteries:

- the two carotids running up in the neck on either side of the windpipe (they provide the pulses you can feel and often see in the throat);
- the basilar artery running up into the head from the front of the spinal cord (it forms where the spine meets the skull from two arteries, the 'vertebrals', running alongside the spine).

The blood flows from all three of these arteries into a circular artery that nestles around the base of the brain, the 'Circle of Willis'. The arteries into the brain itself arise from this circle.

This means that the brain has a unique arrangement for its blood supply. The Circle of Willis protects the brain's circulation from disease of the arteries below it. If one carotid, for example, is badly diseased, and the flow inside it is blocked, the other two arteries provide the extra flow.

On the other hand, if there are problems, such as a block, in the blood vessels above the circle, then it is more difficult to find ways around them. In younger people, collateral vessels sprouting from arteries on the surface of the brain may take over - but this choice is unavailable for the older brain.

Trouble in the brain's circulation comes either because there has been a leak of blood from one of the arteries into the brain, or because an artery has been blocked by clot. There are four ways in which this can happen - in two of which there is bleeding and in two, clotting. The next few pages explain how this condition arise, and describes typical cases of each type of stroke.

*Cerebral hemorrhage*

Around a sixth of strokes are caused by bleeding into the brain. These 'cerebral hemorrhages' are usually the result of years of uncontrolled high blood pressure, aggravated by cigarette smoking. Constant exposure to high blood pressure (hypertension) causes the walls of small arteries to thicken, as a protective response to the pressure within. As we age, however, fatty deposits in these same walls produce weak spots.

The unequal struggle between the defensive thickening and the fatty degeneration has to end with something giving way - and that is the wall of the artery. When it ruptures, blood is forced into the brain tissues under pressure and the damage begins.

As the brain is a relatively soft organ entirely enclosed in a hard case, the skull, the expanding pool of blood not only damages the tissue at the site of bleeding but puts extreme pressure on the rest of the brain. The result is first a severe headache and then a fast lapse into unconsciousness. If the bleeding does not stop, or is not quickly controlled, then recovery is unlikely.

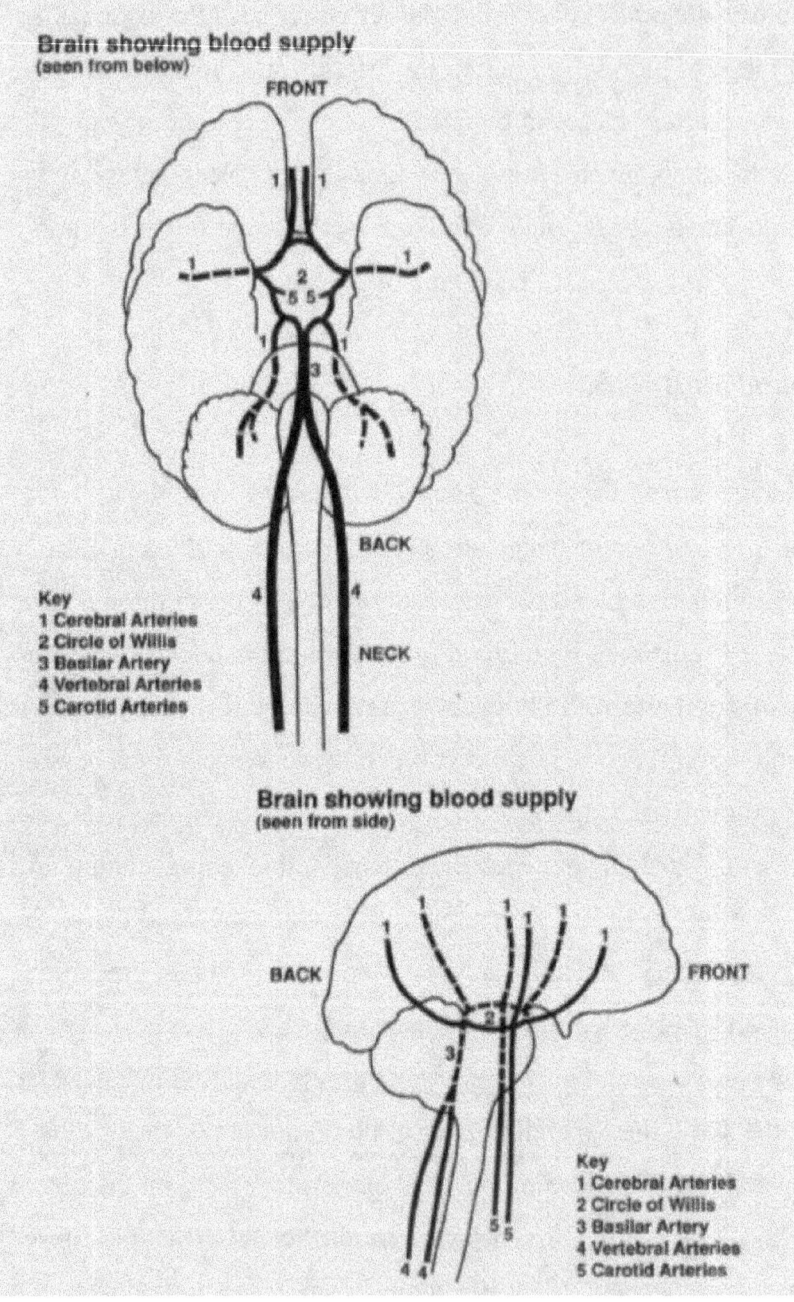

**Brain showing blood supply**
(seen from below)

FRONT

Key
1 Cerebral Arteries
2 Circle of Willis
3 Basilar Artery
4 Vertebral Arteries
5 Carotid Arteries

BACK

NECK

**Brain showing blood supply**
(seen from side)

BACK

FRONT

Key
1 Cerebral Arteries
2 Circle of Willis
3 Basilar Artery
4 Vertebral Arteries
5 Carotid Arteries

Why does smoking matter? There is plenty of evidence that cigarette smoking accelerates the process of fatty degeneration of the cerebral arteries, so that smokers of either sex multiply their chances of stroke many-fold, and especially so if they are also hypertensive.

*Arnold Graham* was 69 when he first visited his doctor. A fiercely independent widower who lived alone, he had to be persuaded to do so by his son who had found him in tears one morning. He had had headaches every morning for the last week or so, he said.
They were becoming worse, lasting longer, and filled his whole head, the pain coming in waves like a beating pulse.
Mr Graham's doctor was alarmed to find that his blood pressure was hugely raised, that he could hardly see, even with his spectacles (this, too, was a new symptom) and to hear, on further questioning, that he had had an attack of weakness in his right arm earlier in the day that had 'passed off'. However, the doctor found that the grip of his right hand was weaker than that of his left - yet he was right handed.
This was enough for the doctor to start him on blood pressure lowering treatment straight away, and to admit him direct from the surgery to hospital. The doctor assumed that he was heading for a stroke in the next few hours if his pressure was not kept under strict control.

Mr Graham was lucky. Intensive treatment for his blood pressure not only helped him to avoid a stroke, it also cured his headaches and brought his vision back to normal within hours. The strength in his right hand took longer to return, but he is now fully recovered and enjoying his 75th year. He still takes tablets to control his blood pressure, but he has stopped smoking - which, until his near-stroke, was his only vice. Instead, he now has an occasional beer – maybe four times a week - as a treat, with his doctor's blessing!

Not everyone is as lucky as Mr Graham. Cerebral hemorrhages do occasionally hit people without warning. Sufferers describe the feeling as if 'someone has hit me, hard, on the head', or as a 'sudden, intense pain, as if my head will burst'. They also complain of being very dizzy, before they lapse into unconsciousness.

However, most cerebral hemorrhages are preceded by warning signs - signs that should raise anyone's suspicions that something is going wrong, and that are ignored at your peril. The first is headache. A throbbing headache that wakens you in the mornings, that seems deep inside the skull, that does not respond to the usual painkillers, and has appeared for the first time in later middle life or beyond, must be presumed to be associated with high blood pressure until proved otherwise.

Unfortunately, headaches are not a feature of many cases of hypertension, so that if you don't have them, you can't assume that you are free of risk. The only way to be sure that your blood pressure is normal is to have it checked.

Other indications that the blood pressure is out of control are dizziness, failing eyesight, and increasing breathlessness on exertion

- such as climbing stairs or walking up a slope. Many people see these signs simply as a part of normal ageing, and don't wish to bother their doctors with them. That can be a big mistake: it is natural to grow old with all one's senses reasonably intact. If your quality of life has suddenly deteriorated, do see your doctor. So much can be done today, not just to control blood pressure safely, but to combine that with a great improvement in one's pleasure in living. That applies as much to ninety-year-olds as to those in their fifties!

One organ that tolerates high blood pressure badly is the kidney. After years of hypertension, kidneys begin to lose their ability to concentrate urine. Sufferers need to rise every night, sometimes more than once, to empty their bladders. Don't ignore this symptom: if it is caused by high blood pressure, controlling it can help the kidney to excellent recovery and at the same time ward off a potential stroke. In any case, don't assume that this too is just a sign of the ageing process. The kidneys do become a little less efficient with age, but not so much as to make regular night walks to the toilet the norm.

The other organ most obviously affected by high blood pressure is the heart. It responds to the extra work it has to do by enlarging. This is fine to begin with but there comes a time, after years of coping with extra pressure, when it begins to fail. It is unable to continue to drive the blood efficiently around the body. These shows up in several ways: people with hypertensive heart failure feel generally weak and lethargic. They become easily breathless with very little exercise, and the ankles and feet may swell.

Although these symptoms are directly due to the failing heart, they are indirect pointers in the high blood pressure patient to possible impending stroke. Uncontrolled high blood pressure is virtually always present in people who have a cerebral hemorrhage, but in fact it more often leads to death from heart attack than from stroke. It is a matter, sadly, of 'if the one does not get you, the other will!'

Happily, the risk of both heart attack and cerebral hemorrhage can be greatly diminished by bringing the blood pressure into the normal range, using modem medicines. This is almost always relatively easily achieved, so that people experiencing these unpleasant symptoms, and frightened of what may be in store for them, can look forward to many more years of useful and enjoyable life.

Subarachnoid hemorrhage

Cerebral hemorrhage is the end result of years of hypertension and blood vessel disease. It usually affects people in late middle age and beyond. It can be prevented, and the fact that there are many fewer cases of hemorrhagic stroke now than in the past is the consequence of recent improvements in preventive medicine and in lifestyles in general.

However, there is one form of hemorrhagic stroke that occurs in much younger people, is less easy to predict and is not associated with high blood pressure. This is 'subarachnoid hemorrhage'.

The subarachnoid space is the area between the surface of the brain and the membrane around it which acts as a framework for the blood vessels, such as the Circle of Willis. The meshwork of vessels in this enveloping membrane is spidery in appearance - hence the name, the arachnoid.

When vessels in the arachnoid leak or burst, the blood oozes around the surface of the brain, putting pressure on the brain at the site of the leak, and raising the pressure, generally, inside the head.
The effect is very similar to that of a cerebral hemorrhage.

The commonest cause of a subarachnoid hemorrhage is a 'berry aneurysm', usually placed on the Circle of Willis at the point of one of its branches into the brain.

Aneurysms are balloon-like pouches arising from the side of an artery. Because they are thin and fragile, they easily burst under pressure. Called 'berry' aneurysms because of their shape and color (at operation they look just like a ripe redcurrant), they form at a weak spot in the wall of the vessel. Normally, in the walls of arteries, there is a thick layer of tough muscle and elastic tissue. This is deficient at spots where aneurysms form, so that the pressure inside blows out the wall, much like the bleb of inner tube that forms through a weak spot in the wall of an old bicycle tire.

It is thought that the tendency to have a berry aneurysm is laid down before birth when the blood vessels are formed. However, leaks from aneurysms are unusual before early adulthood. Peak ages for subarachnoid hemorrhages are from 20 to 40.

*Karen Johnston* was 24 when she had her first headache. It came on after a game of squash and she put it down at first to her just being exhausted and lacking in sugar. A hot sweet tea didn't help, however, and when she found that she couldn't see properly she spoke about it to her boyfriend.

He was alarmed, because she was squinting and one eyelid was drooping. She also had a very stiff neck, and by this time had double vision. Her friend rang her doctor, who wasted no time.

He had her admitted straight to the local neurosurgery unit. By the time she reached the center, she was semi-conscious.

Only a few years ago, Karen's fate from this point onwards would have been a matter of chance. The only treatment the hospital could have provided was life support, and medical treatment to try to relieve the high pressure inside the head. Emergency surgery to stop the bleeding and remove the aneurysm had a very high fatality rate - so high that it was no longer attempted in most centers.

Yet not operating also carried very high risks: one third of all cases of subarachnoid hemorrhage died in the first 24 hours, another third recovered, but with severe long-term disability, and only around a third of cases like Karen's recovered well, to anywhere near the fitness before the hemorrhage. Many of those who recovered to consciousness in the few days after their hemorrhage then had another bleed and died from this second catastrophe.

Today, people like Karen are much more fortunate. The use of the drug nimodipine has brought about a revolution in the early treatment of subarachnoid hemorrhage. Exactly how this treatment works is outside the scope of this book, but it is enough for the moment that it was used in her case to allow the surgeons to operate early to stop the bleeding and to remove the aneurysm.

Within 48 hours she was back to near her normal self, fully conscious and with full movement and sensation in all her limbs. Karen was relatively fortunate. She was hardly lucky, of course, to have had a 'subarachnoid' in the first place, but she was fortunate in that her condition was recognized so early and that she could be brought to a specialist unit and treated so quickly.

In subarachnoid hemorrhage, hours of delay mean a considerable difference to the ultimate chance of survival in a reasonable state. The Danes and Swedes, who have pioneered the modern management of cases of subarachnoid hemorrhage, have a country-wide emergency system, so that any general practitioner who suspects one can summon a special 'squad' that will admit the patient straight into the nearest neurosurgery unit, where surgery to stop the bleeding and relieve the pressure on the brain is started as soon as possible.

This system has brought subarachnoid patients into specialist care up to 48 hours sooner than before, often within one or two hours of the first symptoms. The results have been amazing - the Danes and Swedes have cut their subarachnoid death rates from around 50 per cent to below ten per cent. Just as important, those who do recover do so much more completely, with much less handicap, than before.

*cerebral thrombosis and embolus*

Most strokes are not caused by either form of hemorrhage. 'Thromboses' or 'emboli' within the cerebral arteries are much more common, causing more than three quarters of all strokes.

A thrombus is a clot of blood arising within a blood vessel that blocks the flow through it. An embolus is a piece that has broken from a clot 'upstream' (near the heart) and has been swept into a smaller artery that then becomes blocked by it.

Although the mechanisms are different, the end result is the same: the part of the brain beyond the blocked artery is deprived of its blood supply, and is damaged. If the flow of blood is not turned on again soon, the damage becomes permanent.

In the recent past - until the mid-1960s - medical students were taught that it was possible, from taking a careful history and examining the patient, to distinguish between the different causes of stroke (hemorrhagic, thrombotic or embolic) at the bedside.

Now we know differently. Once a stroke has happened, it is almost impossible to tell for sure what has caused it without hospital tests. The signs and symptoms of stroke - blurring of consciousness, weakness or paralysis of a limb, paralysis of one side of the face, squint, loss of speech and double vision among them - are the same, regardless of the underlying mechanism. They are the result of the damage to the brain, whether it has been caused by hemorrhage or by a clot.

The important point about trying to identify the cause of a stroke is to do so before it happens, not afterwards. For there are often very strong indicators that a stroke is imminent, and if they are recognized early enough the stroke can be prevented, or at the least postponed for some years.

The commonest of these warning signs are 'transient ischemic attacks', or TIAs. 'Ischemia' is simply a medical word for lack of blood flow (the red pigment of blood is 'haem') to an organ. In TIA, the flow of blood to a part of the brain is interrupted for a few seconds. Depending on the area affected, the sufferer can lose, say, the feeling or strength in a limb, feel dizzy and almost pass out, or have a sudden, but temporary, loss of vision.

TIAs pass off very quickly, leaving their victim relieved that they have gone, perhaps a little panicky, but otherwise back to normal. Often, sadly, they do not do any more about them, hoping that they will not return, or at any rate, will never get any worse. They are frightened to seek help, because they fear that they will learn what they already suspect, that they are heading for a stroke. It is understandable that many people just do not wish to have their fears confirmed - but it is also wrong, because their doctors can usually take many practical steps to help ward off the threat.

The vast majority of TIAs are caused by 'showers' of small emboli being flushed through the brain circulation. As they reach the smaller arteries near the brain surface, their bulk briefly blocks the flow, until they are squeezed through the narrowest part of the circulation and back into the venous system that returns the blood to the heart.

These small emboli usually arise from thrombosis that have formed in the carotid arteries in the neck, or perhaps in the heart itself. It is why they form, and what can be done about them, that matters to potential stroke victims.

People with TIAs, and potential thrombo-embolic stroke victims, all have fatty degeneration of their arteries. Many, but not all, have had high blood pressure for years. Very many of the men, and virtually all of the women, have been relatively heavy smokers.

Many, too, have high blood cholesterol levels, are overweight, and eat and drink too well but not too wisely.

The thrombi which have 'thrown off' their emboli to cause their TIAs have formed on sites inside the main arteries from the heart where the fatty degeneration is severe. Instead of the normal smooth inner surface, the blood has to flow over 'plaques' of fatty deposits, full of cholesterol crystals. The eddy currents caused by the irregularity in the vessel wall promotes the start of clotting, presumably in a futile attempt to smooth down the surface and ease the flow of blood over it.

From then on, the process is a vicious circle. The clot narrows the channel through which the blood has to flow, the obstruction worsens, and the eddies created beyond the obstruction cause more clots to form. The body's defenses then try to remove the clot, which breaks up into emboli that are then swept away to smaller vessels. If the main clot is in the carotid artery in the neck, then the likely spot for the embolus to find a niche for itself is the main artery to the middle section of the brain - the middle cerebral artery. As this serves the part of the brain that controls limb movement and sensation, there is weakness and numbness in the appropriate limb. If it is just a small embolus passing through, then the symptoms are transient. However, if it is too big to be processed by the clot dissolving mechanisms in the blood or to pass through the brain circulation back into the main veins, then it will stick there. That is when a TIA becomes a stroke.

*The key to prevention*

Why does the blood clot in the first place? Understanding this is the key to preventing a thrombo-embolic stroke. How we live greatly influences our risks of stroke.

Let's take a typical case history:

Jane Guthrie was in her mid-seventies. She had always enjoyed her food, so that over the years she had put on considerable weight. Not to put too fine a point on it, she was fat. She also liked her drink: three whiskies in a day 'kept her going' , and 'kept her husband company'. As she was never drunk, she saw no reason to cut down. She would have been shocked if anyone had thought her to be alcoholic.

She also smoked. She admitted to twenty cigarettes a day, but she bought more than a dozen packs a week, and her longsuffering husband did not indulge.

Her obesity had also given her mild diabetes: her doctor tried to help her lose weight - crucial to the health of a fat diabetic – but to no avail. She had got to the age of 76, she said, without caring about her figure and she wasn't going to start now.

This description of Mrs Guthrie is perhaps a bit harsh. If it suggests an unlikeable, unfeminine woman, it could not be further from the truth. She had a great sense of humor, took a lively interest in current affairs and politics, played bridge - by all accounts very well and finished The Times crossword every day.

Her good-natured banter with her husband underlined the happy, easy nature of her marriage.

Her troubles started slowly and insidiously. While standing making breakfast one morning she had a fleeting episode of blindness. It lasted only a few seconds, then her vision cleared.

She put the attack down to faintness from lack of food, and decided to ignore it. Just to make sure that it wouldn't bother her again, she took extra jam with her toast!

Over the next few weeks she had several more attacks of blurred vision. They always cleared quickly, but from time to time she also felt quite dizzy and a little nauseated afterwards.

She noticed, too, that her left hand at times felt weaker and colder than the right. What eventually drove her to her doctor, however, was that the right side of her face sometimes sagged, so that she dribbled from the corner of her mouth. When this threatened her social life, she felt that she needed advice!

Her doctor was shocked that she had let things go so far. Her blood pressure was too high for comfort, she was three stones overweight, and blood tests showed that her drinking habits had begun to affect her liver. He was sure that she was heading for a stroke, or perhaps a heart attack, unless she changed her ways.

That meant stopping smoking completely, losing the extra weight, drinking less and exercising more.

Even this was not enough, however. Her doctor was convinced that her symptoms were caused by emboli arising from a clot either in her right carotid artery, or perhaps from her heart. So he arranged an urgent outpatient appointment at the local vascular surgery unit, to identify their source and possibly remove it.

Unfortunately, he was too late. The evening before the hospital appointment Mrs Guthrie was at a family party. For a week she had obeyed orders - at least as well as she could. She had cut down on her cigarettes, had eaten less, restricted her drinks to two a day, and had actually taken a walk or two.

So she thought that she might 'let herself off' for the evening and enjoy herself. Her resolve weakened further after the first aperitif. She ate very well, enjoyed several glasses of wine, and finished the meal with a glass or two of her favorite brandy.

She went to bed very happy, full of food and drink, and fell asleep when her head hit the pillow.

Next morning, her husband could not waken her. She was deeply unconscious, had been incontinent, and her limbs felt, in his words, 'floppy and unmanageable'.

She was admitted to hospital with a severe stroke, from which she never fully recovered. Over many weeks, her consciousness returned, but much of her intellect had gone and her personality with it. She did not regain complete movement or sensation in her left arm and leg, and the right side of her face remained slack and twisted. Over the next year she needed constant nursing care and physiotherapy, and much attention from her loving husband. A year later, almost to the day, she had her second stroke, from which she died.

This story, sadly, is all too common. Mrs Guthrie was on the edge of a precipice and that last evening's over-indulgence almost certainly pushed her over. The meal would have pushed up the levels of fats in her blood, the extra alcohol would have pushed up her blood pressure while slowing the circulation, the extra nicotine would have narrowed the small blood vessels and other chemicals in the cigarette smoke would have made her blood much more viscous. All these effects together would have reached their maximum at around three in the morning, when she was in her deepest sleep. The stroke was virtually inevitable. If only she had known earlier the risks she was taking.

Whether Jane's stroke stemmed from a thrombus arising in a cerebral artery, or from an embolus from elsewhere in the circulation, is academic once the stroke has done its damage. What really matters is to recognize the signs of impending stroke beforehand, and to take action on them. Many strokes may be averted, or at least postponed by judicious care or even emergency treatment, if action is taken in time.

If Jane, for example, had seen her doctor immediately after her first bout of blindness, she might well have been offered carotid artery-surgery to remove the initial thrombus. Anti-coagulant drugs may have prevented further clotting, and even as simple a remedy as half an aspirin a day might have done so.

Being more disciplined about her smoking, drinking and eating habits might also have helped, but her doctors would have played this down after the event, as there is no point in adding feelings of guilt to the stress of a catastrophic stroke. There is enough misery after a stroke, for both sufferer and carer, without anyone putting the blame for the stroke entirely on the victim's pre-stroke lifestyle. That said, it has to be admitted that the way we live does greatly influence our risk of stroke.: Anything we do to:

• raise our blood pressures (such as drinking too much alcohol, eating too much salt)

• increase the levels of fats in our circulation (such as consuming too much animal fat, dairy products, or just consuming too much!)

• stimulate the tendency of our blood to clot (such as cigarette smoking) will raise our stroke risk.

Conversely, anything we do to:

• lower our blood pressure (such as taking regular exercise, eating less salt, relaxing more and sleeping well)

• reduce the levels of the wrong form of fats in the blood (by eating more cereals, fruit and vegetables, choosing fish and poultry rather than red meats or dairy products, and just eating less)

• decrease the tendency of blood to clot (such as taking half an aspirin a day and avoiding cigarettes, your own or other people's) will lower your stroke risk.

*Early warning signs*

Most important of all, see your doctor urgently if you start to have symptoms similar to those experienced by Arnold, Karen or Jane. Here is a list of those early warning symptoms that you should see your doctor to have checked:

• early morning headaches that are there on waking

• any severe headache that does not improve with the usual painkillers

• disturbances of vision that clear within a few minutes

• fleeting bouts of weakness, numbness or 'pins and needles' in an arm or leg

• any visual disturbance or faintness linked with turning the head to one side

• bouts of dizziness, faintness or nausea that start for no apparent reason

• short bouts of confusion that clear quickly and completely

• persistent buzzing in the ears not explained by ear problems

It must be said here that none of these symptoms on their own necessarily suggest impending stroke, and that most are usually caused by more minor health problems - migraine, for example. However they all need to be investigated to rule out impending stroke in a small number of people.

Delay in seeking advice is wholly understandable: many people are frightened by what they may find out about themselves, and push their worries to the back of their minds. The extra anxiety often makes them drink, smoke and eat even more - exactly the opposite of what they should be doing!

Yet taking action to prevent a stroke can be so easy, and even pleasurable. Changing to a more physically active life, with new eating habits and better health, can make you feel like a new person. To make the best of the change, you should make it under your doctor's supervision. Doctors will do their utmost to reduce the chances of thrombosis or hemorrhage with medicines and, where necessary, surgery.

Going on your own personal stroke prevention program like this offers you two important bonuses. The first is the kick you will get out of doing something positive to improve your own quality of life. The second is at least as important as preventing a stroke. Most people like Mrs Guthrie who have TIAs do not, in fact, go on to suffer a stroke. They have heart attacks before the stroke occurs. Their illness is symptomatic of general blood vessel disease, which includes fatty degeneration (atheroma) in the coronary arteries that feed the heart. TIAs are even more of a warning of a probable coronary thrombosis (heart attack) than of stroke.

The treatment of TIAs, which includes all the measures described above, will help to fend off a heart attack just as much as it will prevent stroke. So there are two major benefits in taking the one action. More than half of all the deaths before the age of 65 in most developed countries are caused by heart attack and stroke - we can prepare ourselves to avoid them as soon as we are old enough to understand about how to live to give ourselves the best chance of continuing good health.

Even if we have not heeded the healthy living message until the warning signs have appeared, it's never too late to change. There is always something we can do, positively, to help ourselves.

A last word on prevention. Even though many strokes might have been prevented by more sensible living habits, there are people who suffer from them, out of the blue, with no warning, and who have lived healthily and wisely.

There is never any point, once a stroke has occurred, trying to seek blame or to apportion guilt. No one, victim or carer, should entertain feelings of guilt, or ask 'Why me?', or ponder over 'what might have been' or 'if only I'd ... '. All these attitudes waste time - valuable time that could be focused on helping the victim back to as near a normal life as possible, or coping as well as possible with any residual disability.

The next chapters describe what happens once a stroke has occurred, how it is managed in hospital, and how family and friends, and the people working in the general practice health care team, can best build on that initial care later in the home.

# 2 The First Few Days

Strokes range in their effects from the very mild - no more than a slight difficulty with speech or a weakness in the fingers - to the disastrous, in which there is fast progress into coma and little hope of recovery.

Most strokes lie somewhere between these two extremes. Many start with a minor disability, then worsen slowly over hours or days.

All minor strokes must be presumed, to begin with, to be such a 'stroke in evolution', so that even if victims are only mildly affected they should be admitted to a specialist stroke unit in hospital without delay. Many families, understandably, would like to keep them at home, on the premise that they can give round-the-clock nursing care and the added benefits that the extra love in home surroundings can offer.

However, this may not be in the best interest of the patient.

Hospitals can offer on-the-spot emergency specialist treatment if there is sudden deterioration; and 24-hour a day professional nursing, combined with expert physiotherapy, must be superior to, say, the most devoted but exhausted wife or husband.

The first few days in hospital are a period of initial examination, investigation and assessment. The first examination will include a detailed study of the nervous system: if the patient is conscious, this will include testing of:

- the strength and co-ordination of movement in the limbs and face

- all aspects of sensation, which includes touch, pressure, blunt and sharp pain, sensitivity to heat and cold, and the sense of position in space
- the special senses of vision, hearing, taste and smell
- orientation in space and time (knowledge of where he is and what day and year it is)
- understanding and intellect.

This last is important, not only to assess any stroke-induced loss, but also as a baseline for any improvement or deterioration later. It is difficult, too, because strokes can cause problems with hearing, word memory and speech that can complicate assessment of true intellectual loss. Many people with strokes understand more than they initially seem to - and one of the reasons for our modern active approach to rehabilitation after the first days is to bring out the best in all of them.

If the patient is in coma, it is important to define the level of unconsciousness. Reflex reactions to stimuli, such as the way the pupils respond to light, the knee jerk and the sole-stroke responses, and assessment of the tone in the affected muscles, help the doctor assess the extent of the brain damage.

Use of an ophthalmoscope allows doctors to examine the optic nerve inside the eye. This nerve carries the sensation of sight from the retina to the brain, and appears swollen if the brain is under high pressure: this can be an indication for emergency action to prevent further brain damage. High pressure inside the brain can be reduced very quickly by an infusion into the veins (a drip) of a concentrated solution of a form of sugar (mannitol) that sucks fluid from the tissues into the circulation.

Repeating all these examinations over the following few days help to define the extent of recovery and deterioration. It can be days, weeks or even, though rarely, months, before recovery towards consciousness starts: the first signs of such recovery are subtle changes in the reflexes.

Other investigations aim to find the cause of the stroke. The simplest are among the routine tests of any physical examination - the pulse, blood pressure and use of the stethoscope.

An irregular pulse may be one sign of fatty degenerative heart and artery disease - atheroma. That points to a thrombosis, either in the heart itself or in the carotid arteries, from which an embolus might have reached the brain. Measures to deal with such clots, such as anticoagulant drugs (heparin, warfarin or even aspirin) may be prescribed. Drugs to make the heart's rhythm more regular (antiarrhythmics) may also be considered. In rare cases, a thrombus in a carotid artery may be considered so life-threatening that surgery (endarterectomy) is needed to remove it.

Blood pressure measurement is an essential in all stroke cases. On admission it can be at any level: the damage to the brain may have caused circulation collapse, so that it is unrecordably low, and the patient is in shock. On the other hand, the stroke may be the end result of years of high blood pressure (hypertension), and the pressure may still be unacceptably high. A normal blood pressure reading may not necessarily be reassuring: in those who were hypertensive before their stroke, it could be a sign of shock. It is important, therefore, to let the hospital doctors know, if possible, what the usual blood pressure was before the stroke.

The stethoscope is needed to assess how well the heart and circulation are doing. An irregular heart may confirm suspicions of a thrombo-embolic cause. More than that, the sound of a murmur over a carotid artery points to an area of narrowing, either by atheroma or thrombus, this may need urgent attention. Any degree of heart failure will be spotted from the sound of fluid in the bases of the lungs.

If there is any doubt about the heart, two more investigations are needed: an electrocardiogram and an echocardiogram. The first will define the nature of any abnormal rhythm, so that the correct drug treatment can be chosen. The second gives the physician a moving picture of how the heart is beating: it can identify a thrombus within one chamber of the heart that might be the source of an embolus.

Other body systems must also be checked. Poorly controlled diabetes puts people at higher risk than normal of stroke, so blood levels of glucose, which are high in diabetes, are measured. Rarely, strokes may result from *low* blood glucose, a condition arising from tumors of the pancreas. In either case, the first concern is to correct the blood abnormality and to return the glucose levels to the normal range. This can be dramatic with, on occasion, patients in near comatose states recovering consciousness over a few hours. The task then is to deal with the diabetes or the pancreatic mass.

Very rarely, stroke can be the first sign of tumor in the brain. The commonest source of such tumors is a primary cancer in the lung, so that this will also be ruled out by careful examination and X-ray, if necessary.

At the same time a series of tests to identify the physical cause and site of the stroke are undertaken. Where an aneurysm is suspected, special X-rays (angiograms) outline the circulation in the carotid arteries and Circle of Willis. A computerized tomography (CAT scan), in which a series of X-rays is built up into a complete 'map' of the inside of the skull, may be needed to identify areas of brain damage from hemorrhage or thrombosis. Some hospitals use injections of 'trace' amounts of radio-isotopes to identify the areas of loss of blood flow within the brain.

The point of all these tests is to make sure that if there is a way that medical or surgical treatment can ease the damage done by the stroke, it will be found. However, for most stroke victims, the important point of these first few days is whether they are beginning to recover or are sinking into a deepening coma. Despite the use of modern treatments to reduce the pressure within the brain, for most stroke victims recovery from these first few days depends most on the extent and site of the initial thrombosis or hemorrhage. If the damage is too extensive, or has affected a critical part of the brain, then the chance of recovery is remote, regardless of treatment. However, if the patient's condition becomes stable in the first two to three days, there is usually considerable scope for recovery, and it can be helped on by skilled medical and nursing care and physiotherapy. As the high pressure inside the brain subsides and the swelling lessens, the brain cells in the penumbra - the area around the centrally affected site - recover to a more normal state, and consciousness begins to return, along with movement and sensation. It is from this crucial time onwards that active treatment to return the patient as much as possible to normal should start. That usually means transfer to a specialized stroke unit in which doctors, nurses, physiotherapists, occupational therapists, speech therapists, teachers and, most important, the patients and their relatives themselves, are all actively - and energetically - involved in the task of rehabilitation. Before that can be done, however, the extent of the patient's problems must be very carefully assessed and detailed plans made to tackle them. To understand why this is needed the handicaps arising from stroke must be explained, This is done in the next chapter.

# 3 The Aftermath of Stroke

The type of disability that a stroke leaves behind depends very precisely on the area of brain affected, How we move, feel, see, talk, hear, smell and think depends on the integrity of different parts of the surface of the brain - the cerebral cortex. Remove the blood supply to that part of the brain, and its specific function is lost.

As each half of the brain is served by its own main arteries arising from its half of the Circle of Willis, strokes almost always affect sites in only one side of the brain, For it to affect both sides, it would have to be massive, and almost certainly non-survivable. So the effects of most strokes are one-sided - either the left or the right halves of the body are affected, but not both,

Areas of cerebral cortex differ, too, in their importance. For example, there are areas of the front part of the cortex that appear to be relatively inactive, in that they can be lost without causing obvious handicap. On the other hand, even a small stroke affecting the area immediately behind the frontal area can cause paralysis (hemiplegia), or loss of sensation (hemiparesis), of the opposite side of the body and of the same side of the head. Often, the two go together.

Distressing as loss of power and sensation in limbs obviously is, they are not a complete description of hemiplegia and hemiparesis. Immediately after a stroke, the affected limbs are initially loose and flaccid in tone. But within hours, they become stiffer, or 'spastic'.

This means that the affected muscles tend to contract on their own at the slightest hint of stretching. The reflexes in the elbow, wrist, knee and ankle become exaggerated. When the sole of the foot is stroked, the big toe stretches upwards and the other toes tend to fan out, which is quite different from the normal reaction of curling downwards.

This spasticity poses an immediate problem for the carers, one that persists throughout life where recovery is incomplete. The affected limbs must be regularly stretched over the full range of their joint movements. If they are not, the limb will curl up and the muscles contract. Over the next few months, if physiotherapy is neglected, the deformity will become irreversible.

Hemiparesis, too, is not simply a loss of feeling. A stroke leaves its victims with no idea of the position of their affected arm and leg: in fact they may be wholly unaware of that half of their body. It can take some persuasion for some patients to accept that they still possess their 'missing' limbs! This clearly produces difficulties for their nurses and other carers because, in the initial days at least, they are unable to co-operate with the simplest of instructions.

As victims of hemiparesis also find it impossible to identify by feel everyday objects, such as pens, cutlery and keys, the size of the task of retraining can be imagined. What is essential is that it should be started as early as possible - preferably as soon as the acute emergency has ended and obvious signs of recovery have begun to appear.

Strokes affecting the cortex at the back of the brain may result in blindness. The distribution of the nerves leading from the eyes to the brain is such that, when a stroke occurs on one side of this part of the cortex, the vision is lost from the same half of each eye. That means that half the victim's field of vision is lost. As the right half of each eye sees the left half of the field of vision, and vice versa, loss of the 'visual' cortex in the right half of the brain means seeing nothing to the left of the midline. The opposite obtains, of course, for a left sided stroke. This is hemianopia.

Surprisingly, perhaps, many people with hemianopia find it difficult to describe. They may not even know they have it. There is no black cloud across half the old field of vision: it is often only when sufferers undergo vision testing that it is diagnosed. Obviously, everyone who has recovered from stroke must have their visual fields tested to rule out hemianopia before they start driving again. Not seeing what is coming from one side, and not even knowing that you are blind on that side, is, needless to say, very dangerous!

Serious as loss of movement, sensation and vision are, they are not always the worst stroke-related disabilities. Right-handed people who have right-sided strokes - that is, the right arm and leg, and left side of the face, are affected - have problems in the left side of the brain. This also happens to house a small, but very important 'center of communications' called Broca's area. If this is damaged, then the abilities to speak, write, read and understand language are affected. In left-handed people, a left-sided stroke has the same effect.

The medical name for this is aphasia, or dysphasia. Depending on the precise site of the stroke, aphasia can result from a block to the processing of information entering the 'center', or from an inability to express information to the outside world. In severe cases, obviously more difficult to manage, both understanding and expression are affected. The result is that some stroke victims cannot speak at all, and others are still fluent in language, but what they say appears to be nonsense.

Another speech disturbance, apraxia (or dysarthria), arises not from damage to the communication center, but to the part of the cortex that controls the muscles of speech in the voice box (the larynx), the tongue, lips and the soft palate. In this case, language is understood, but the difficulty is in the mechanics of its expression.

Such patients also have difficulty in swallowing, so they are at risk of choking when they try to eat.

Naturally, when movement, sensation, and vision are faulty, and the patient is aphasic, many other social functions taken for granted when healthy will also be affected. The three Rs are among the skills that may have to be learned all over again. Apart from the visual disability, which makes reading difficult in the first place, some strokes leave people with alexia, a condition in which it is not possible to understand words written across the page. Oddly, some sufferers can understand words if the letters are printed vertically, a finding that can sometimes be used to help retraining, provided it is started soon after the stroke.

Alexia may disappear quickly and completely but for some recovery is partial, and for a few the condition is permanent. Patients who have read more before their stroke are said to have a better chance of recovery from alexia, but it is difficult to predict in the first few days the chances of a particular person's recovery. Along with alexia there is agraphia, or inability to write. Recovery from this, too, varies from person to person. Perhaps saddest of all such sufferers are the musicians who can no longer write or understand written music. Some people retain the ability to write, but find the choice of the correct word for the meaning they are trying to express impossible. They may have lost the ability to spell, or repeat or miss out letters. Aphasia can be associated with loss of mathematical skills such as addition and subtraction. Recognition of the numbers themselves may be lost. However, as the recovery from stroke progresses this usually returns, often very fully. A schoolteacher who specialized in mathematics was unable to work because of a stroke that left him unable to comprehend single-figure addition sums: within two years he was able to teach again. Of course, not all recoveries are so spectacular: much depends on the previous development of the skill that has been lost, and the determination of both patient and carers to fight on. All these difficulties: aphasia, alexia, agraphia and loss of numeracy, stem, as explained above, from strokes in the left half of the brain in right-handed people, and in the right half of the brain in left handers. When the trouble is on the opposite side, skills in receiving and expressing communications are left untouched. There is still hemiplegia and hemiparesis, but life is much easier.

However, even this form of stroke has its extra difficulties over and above those of paralysis and loss of sensation. In right handers (of course, the opposite is the case for left handers), the right half of the brain is responsible for judgment of perspective, distance, shape and the inter-relationship of objects in our immediate environment.

Life can still be very difficult - but in a completely different way. The two halves of the brain have quite different functions. The half on the opposite side of our 'handedness', as we have seen, controls movement, feeling and co-ordination of such things as speech.

The half of the brain on the same side as our handedness, however, has a much more subtle job to do. It is responsible for all sorts of judgmental decisions, such as perception of perspective, of distance, shape, position in space, and the inter-relationship of objects in our immediate environment.

This means that a stroke on the same side of the brain as our strongest hand - left side for left handers and right side for right handers - has its particular difficulties. What were routine activities, like eating, applying make-up, combing hair, shaving, tooth brushing, washing and dressing, are now very difficult or even impossible.

Many people with this form of stroke do not fully realize, or they even deny, the extent of their difficulties and carry on regardless with what they are attempting to do. This can lead at its simplest to (say) putting on clothes outside in, but more seriously to high risks of domestic accidents. It is vital, therefore, that those caring for such stroke victims do not underestimate their difficulties.

The fact that speech is intact does not rule out the need for special help in re-training the patient in organizing his or her everyday tasks. Without such help, life can be as frustrating for the person with left sided stroke as for the one whose right-sided stroke has been complicated by speech difficulties and other problems of communication.

For some people, left-sided strokes are disastrous. Imagine the distress of artists or architects who have lost their sense of perspective and position, who can still draw adequately because the drawing arm and the skill have been unaffected, but whose finished work is essentially a jumbled mass of unrelated objects. They need special attention and sympathy if they are to be helped towards recovery.

Incontinence must also be mentioned here. During the initial period of acute stroke, with some disturbance of consciousness, most patients are incontinent of urine and some are also faecally incontinent. This is because, while the higher brain functions are temporarily suspended, the bladder and bowel empty automatically when they become full.

For the vast majority of stroke victims, this period quickly passes and full continence returns within days. In the meantime, however, a catheter may have to be passed to drain the urine, mainly to keep the patient comfortable and dry. Very rarely, the incontinence does not recover and arrangements must be made for long-term care. This will be organized in hospital, well before the person is discharged home. In most areas today, there are special home incontinence services that help the family and the patient to cope successfully with the problem.

For people unused to dealing with incontinence, the prospect is both frightening and distasteful but the modern aids are both easy to work with and as acceptable aesthetically as possible in the circumstances. Learning to deal with incontinence is a challenge, but it is not insuperable and it is surprising how quickly it can become routine and of little bother. Nowadays, every district hospital has a specialist incontinence unit. If the problem persists, then referral to this unit for detailed assessment and planning of its eventual management can help very much.

All the problems described in this chapter are essentially physical, are relatively easy to spot, and can be readily understood. Most can be greatly improved, and where improvement is limited, some way can usually be found to cope with them. More difficult to define are the effects on the patient's psyche. Stroke can understandably alter the patient's mood: depression is a very common and serious complication of stroke. Relatives are often faced, too, with changes in personality and a drop in intellect that can be real or apparent.

These changes in the mental state, and how they can be faced, are discussed in the next chapter.

# 4 Mood, Mind and Personality

It would be astonishing, to say the least, if there were no psychological changes after an illness as devastating as stroke. Among them are depression, anxiety, and even guilt, as people often think, usually mistakenly, that they have brought their illness upon themselves.

Yet this is by no means the whole story. The brain is also responsible for mood and personality, as well as intellect, and any damage to it can cause profound changes beyond the natural reaction to the change in the patient's physical condition. It is very common for relatives of stroke sufferers to be more upset by the apparent change in their personality than by the physical disability.

In the first few days, it is absolutely normal for the sufferer to react to the stroke with depression, irritation and frustration. In fact, it would be abnormal for it to be otherwise, and even a matter of concern to the medical staff. This initial phase, however, soon passes. Most recover well psychologically as the physical condition improves and the professional help brings comfort and reassurance. However, in a few people, stroke does alter the way they think and the way they react to circumstances. Some with left-sided strokes may not realize that they have been severely disabled by their illness, so that they see themselves as still able to function physically in every way normally, even though they are paralyzed down one side. One way to test this is to ask them if they can drive.

Most patients will admit that this is no longer possible: some will cheerfully claim that they still can, and do not see their paralysis as a problem. Although this may in the short term be a benefit for the patient's own feeling of well-being, it can be a source of distress for his or her family who have to cope with the real circumstances.

More common is the opposite reaction. Many stroke victims become more inward-looking, less sociable, less inclined to start any communication between themselves and their carers. To their wives or husbands, in particular, this is a shock. Confronted with a miserable, pessimistic spouse fearing for the future, the temptation is for the whole family to feel likewise, with disastrous consequences for any thought of rehabilitation.

The only way to face this reaction is to be optimistic. Once you are aware that this is not an inevitable, irreversible result of the stroke, but an understandable reaction to it that can be reversed, then it can be dealt with. The whole family must assume that inside the 'changed' person is the old personality trying to break through again, and the process can be pushed forward if those around him share all the family news, build up his confidence, and help him to a more positive view of his own future. Above all, people like this need to feel they still have the respect of, and are much needed by, the rest of their family.

Inactivity in a stroke patient can be as distressing as emotional disturbance. In the early days and weeks after a stroke, many people simply seem to lose interest in life. They never initiate conversation, take no interest in what is going on around them, and when brought into any family activity, their concentration quickly flags. They are easily tired, so that they never finish, and often never find the energy to start, simple jobs that they may wish to do or have been set.

This inactivity is only partly due to tiredness: it may also be a way of avoiding the stress of trying to make decisions - something new stroke victims find very difficult, and will avoid where possible.

The answer is a two-fold approach. Some part of the day, say the mid-afternoon, should be set aside as a rest period. For the rest of the time, they should be encouraged to make their own decisions about their everyday lives, such as their choice of clothes and how to spend the evening, and be brought into family discussions and decisions.

One feature of stroke that often greatly upsets the family is a change in emotional reactions. As children, we cry very easily when we are hurt or frustrated: we are taught to lose this response as we grow up. In stroke this self-control is often lost, so that the victim may burst into tears at the slightest provocation, often quite inappropriately. Such outbursts are not a sign of depression or even of distress.

They are more likely to be tears of embarrassment and frustration because the emotions cannot be kept under control. There may be elements of fear, anger and a sense of loss behind them, none of which can be expressed in any other way but tears.

The same person can suddenly switch from tears to laughter, again for no obvious reason. The laughter may be so uncontrolled that it sounds almost maniacal - an experience that is even more disturbing than tears for family and friends. An occasional outburst of swearing will also shock, especially when it comes from someone who has always been careful about his or her language.

All these bizarre behaviors must be met with the understanding that they are outside the patient's control. The best way to deal with them is to ignore them, and continue to converse with him in a normal, calm, objective way. If they are provoked by something that is clearly the source of frustration, then the carer must try to help him through it.

If such outbursts become so common that they are almost the norm in relationships between patient and carer, then some action must be taken. There is no point in the carer becoming angry or arguing, although it does no harm when the outburst is over to explain that it is not an acceptable way to behave. Giving way to demands made under emotional stress will not help towards eventual rehabilitation. The carer must strike a balance between sympathy for the plight of the patient and the need to correct obviously antisocial and disturbing behavior.

Much of the abnormal behavior stems from the frustration that arises because three aspects of normal intellect have been disturbed - memory, concentration span and logical thought. In the early recovery period, relatives can be shocked by the victim's apparent considerable loss of intelligence. However, it is often very difficult to differentiate in these early days between real intellectual loss and the emotional depression that follows the patient's realization of his disabilities. The second tends to recover quickly: the first may need months to improve upon and, in fact, may never recover to any great extent.

Loss of memory is a feature of many strokes: it varies from mild - such as a blank few days before the attack - to severe, in which the patient has virtually no memory at all, especially for what has just been happening around him. Memory for events of many years past, however, is usually retained. This is particularly important, as retraining the memory is much easier if it is built upon what is still in the 'store'. It is even easier still if it is conducted in the patient's own home, where the familiarity with the environment lessens any confusion.

Improving the time that the patient can spend in concentrating on a subject - his attention span - is also vital to improving intellectual performance. This, too, is most effectively done in the home, by family and friends who are both encouraging and firm at the same time.

The combination of some loss of intellect, of memory, and of the ability to concentrate, and the difficulty many patients have of coming to terms with and understanding what has happened to them, often leads to confusion. The best way to deal with this is to start early to set up a daily routine that they can feel comfortable with and to bring the confusion out into the open in conversation. By showing that the confusion is understood and that steps are being taken to minimize its causes, much of it will diminish.

This is particularly important for aphasic patients. Carers will be trained by the hospital staff, before the patient arrives home, on how to deal with his or her type and extent of aphasia. It is enough here to state that conversation is vital. It must be normal talking, exactly as before the stroke, with constant encouragement to the patient to return the communication in any way possible. Preferably it should be speech, but if that is impossible then sign language, hand signals, or tapping out messages on a word processor or typewriter keyboard are all excellent substitutes. The important point is that understanding should be established between carer and patient. Once it is, then the confusion will lessen and the new understanding can be used as a springboard for further progress in rehabilitation.

Two other vital points about communications must be made here. First, carers should never assume that because stroke victims are unable to converse they cannot understand what is being said around them. So *never* talk about them to others when they are present. It is most distressing for them, making them feel less than human, and will almost certainly delay any potential return towards normality.

The second point-is that, in speaking to stroke patients, there is no need either to shout (strokes do not make you deaf) or to address them as if they were children. This also demeans and insults adults who retain their ability to think but who cannot express themselves adequately.

After a stroke some people will never be the same as they were: there may be residual physical disabilities and intellectual and other psychological and memory deficits. However, with a correct approach many of these deficits and handicaps can be made good or at least considerably improved. The following chapters describe the ways in *which this* is now being achieved.

# 5 The Way Back

The immediate aftermath
of a stroke is very frightening and depressing for relatives and
friends. Sitting by the bedside of an unconscious, paralyzed,
obviously very sick person, it is difficult to accept that he or she
might ever recover to full consciousness or mobility.

Yet it does happen and the process of recovery starts very soon after
the stroke. When the hemorrhage or thrombosis has been brought
under control, and the high pressure within the brain subsides,
consciousness and movement begin to return within hours.

It is the task of the hospital staff - doctors, nurses and
physiotherapists in the first place, and occupational and speech
therapists later - to ensure that the initial progress is as fast and
complete as possible.

After that, it is the family's turn to continue the process *with* the help
of the home health care team.

It is natural to ask, in these first few days, about the prospects of the
patient. Will he recover at all? How much recovery is likely?
What will be the residual handicap? How long will it be before we
know the final extent of the handicap?

The answers to these questions are never simple. Some people
recover remarkably from the most severe strokes, particularly if they
are young. Others remain relatively severely handicapped and make
little progress. It is difficult to predict what will happen in a
particular patient. However, there are general *rules* that govern the
chances of recovery in most strokes:

- The worse the initial effects of the stroke, the longer it is before recovery is complete.

- Strokes that start slowly, and worsen only over several hours, (that start as 'strokes in evolution'), are usually less severe than sudden collapse into unconsciousness, and recovery from them is faster and often more complete.

- Recovery depends to some extent on previous intelligence, education and character. The brighter and more forceful and active a person is before a stroke, the better is the probable recovery.

- Emotional problems such as depression or an anxiety state before a stroke are a pointer to poorer than normal recovery.
They may well need special attention after the stroke, by doctors and the various therapists: they may tend to be forgotten in its aftermath, but they will still be an underlying obstacle to more complete recovery.

- Particular skills that the person has had for years are usually less damaged than recently acquired and less well developed skills.
How well the patient recovers depends, of course, largely on the amount of brain damaged by the stroke. However, it also depends greatly on recognition of the need for early and skilful professional help. The sooner treatment is started; the more likely it is to contribute to the fullest possible recovery.

Helping stroke victims to recovery also depends on the attitudes of the carers. It is natural to be sympathetic towards the patient, to do things for him, and to encourage him to rest. In fact, this can often be just the opposite of what is needed. Most patients do far better if they are encouraged to be active and to do as much as possible for themselves. If this leads to confrontation, and even to arguments and emotional scenes, so be it. They are a normal part of the physical and mental rehabilitation that cannot be avoided if the best is to be made of the patient's remaining facilities.

The two main priorities in the early days are to help the patient to become mobile, and to be able to communicate. As muscles begin to recover and he can converse, in whatever way, with friends, relatives and staff, the patient's attitude changes. His fear and misery can turn to optimism and co-operation, and the new, more positive attitude helps to accelerate the improvement. That brings more optimism and with it a beneficial spiral towards better health begins. The better the patient feels the faster will be the recovery. The faster the recovery, the better the patient feels - and so on. This will not happen, however, without considerable effort by everyone involved, including the closest family.

*Getting moving again*

The first priority of all - and the one that seems cruelest to many who are experiencing a stroke, or nursing a stroke patient, for the first time - is to get the patient out of bed as soon as possible after consciousness returns.

Lying in bed can be fatal! First of all, any extended period of immobility greatly reduces muscle power and muscle bulk, even in the muscles not affected by the stroke. It also allows calcium to leak away from the bone, weakening it and increasing the future risk of fracture.

Lying in bed can also let the circulation in the legs and pelvis stagnate, which can lead to thrombosis in the deep veins. The risk of to the lungs, where they can cause sudden death, is very high.

These problems are multiplied in patients who are overweight. Fat people have often been less physically active than normal before their strokes: they are less inclined to move themselves afterwards - and are more difficult to move - than their leaner colleagues. This means that a very special effort has to be made to get fat people moving early: if they stay immobile for long, they will never walk again.

A very strong effort should also be made to make them lose their extra pounds. This can obviously be difficult, when the energy they expend is so small and the appetite is undiminished by the stroke. It is not a matter of going on a diet, but of eating much less than before.

Advice that the patient should become physically active seems, at first, strange to family carers who, because one half of their relative's body cannot move, tend to think that the whole person must be immobile. This initial and understandable feeling must be fought against vigorously. At least half the body's muscles remain within the control of the patient, and can be exercised fully and energetically. The other half, even though paralyzed, must be kept mobile - something that the carers must first organize themselves, and then teach the patient himself to do.

This is not easy for the patient. It is natural for him to feel self pity and to resent, or even rage against, the condition in which he finds himself. A common reaction is to wish to lie in bed, turning against anyone trying to help. This resentment against his condition, the world in general and his carers in particular, is complicated further by his loss of body image. He feels as if he is only half the person he was and may not even be persuaded that he is still a whole human being until he is shown his reflection in a mirror.

At the same time, action must be taken to keep the affected limbs supple and at least passively mobile. If they are not regularly stretched and moved through their whole normal range of positions, they will become contracted and stiff. The affected elbow and wrist bend up, the fingers curl, the knee and ankle straighten out, the head twists to one side, the shoulder droops backwards, the body falls to one side, and the patient becomes twisted, curling up sideways towards his affected side. If he is allowed to remain in this state, recovery of good muscle movement will be impossible, even if the nervous system that serves the affected muscles recovers.

The aim of all stroke treatment from the start, therefore, is to keep the whole body and limbs in as near normal a posture as possible, whether the patient is lying, sitting or being helped to stand.

Every joint should be attended to: the neck, spine, arms and fingers should be straightened, the thigh pushed out sideways and forwards from the hip, with the knee bent and the foot turned upwards. In bed, these positions can be held by strategically placed pillows. This is particularly important when the patient is lying on his or her back, a position not recommended, except for a few minutes at a time to relieve pressure on the skin in other areas. The relatively immobile patient should be placed on one side, changing the side every two hours or so, night and day, to prevent pressure sores.

When lying on the affected side, the affected arm should be gently pulled out straight so that the shoulder blade moves forward. This prevents pressure being placed on the point of the shoulder. The affected thigh should be positioned straight down in line with the trunk, so that the hip joint is not bent, and the knee bent by lifting up the ankle. The affected knee should not be left in the straight position.

When lying on the unaffected side, the 'bad' arm should again be pulled out straight from the shoulder, and a pillow put beneath it to support it. The affected leg should be flexed on the hip just enough to prevent him from turning onto his back, and the knee rested on a pillow. A small cushion under the space between the top of the hip and the ribs will stop the spine from slumping into the bed.

On either side, the head should rest on just enough pillows - usually two - to keep the neck straight. Some patients find it difficult to breathe when lying flat: this can be solved by putting the head of the bed on specially designed non-slip blocks.

The intensity of the contractions in the affected muscles depends greatly on the position in which the patient is lying or sitting. If the head is turned away from the affected side, the muscle tone in the affected limbs increases and the muscles contract. Stroke patients must be encouraged to look towards their affected side - a task that may be difficult, as they often feel that it does not exist and tend to face away from it.

*Shifting position in bed*

The first essential of self-help is for the patient to be able to roll himself from one side to the other in bed. This starts with him holding the weak hand with the good one, and using the good arm to stretch the arms up into the air. This raises the paralyzed shoulder. Turning the head, then the arms, towards the unaffected side shifts the body weight round, so that the torso follows, along with the legs and feet.

At first, the patient will need considerable help just to do this, but he should be encouraged from very early on in his recovery to feel free to switch sides by himself. He, and his carers, must take great care of the affected shoulder during all turning movements. It is very easily damaged, particularly if the arm is pulled or rolled on. And as there is often no sensation in the shoulder, the patient may not know that it has been injured.

Hospital staff will train carers in how to move patients safely, to avoid injuries. One absolute DON'T is to move a patient by placing a hand under his affected arm and lifting. On the paralyzed side, the muscles around the joint can no longer provide resistance to strain, and the shoulder joint is left unprotected. The result can be permanent damage to the joint.

It is in these few early days that the pattern for improvement is established. Many stroke sufferers react very badly to the first efforts to make them mobile. They do not yet understand why they are being 'bullied' and not only resent the help but can actively resist it. This is often the time of the worst emotional outbursts, of raging bad temper and fits of screaming or weeping.

It can be difficult for non-professional carers to carry on at this stage. When everything seems so difficult, even pointless, and all you get for your trouble is anger and abuse rather than gratitude, it is easy either to give up or to become angry and upset yourself.

Do resist either option. The only way to respond is to remember that it is the frustration from the brain damage that is causing the behavior change, and to keep up the good work. Be firm and patient, but carry on regardless with the retraining process. As your patient begins to sense an improvement, the resentment usually fades, co-operation begins, and confidence and hope start to grow.

*Sitting up*

The next step is for him to sit up. Early on, the carers may have to do all the work of moving the patient themselves. To begin with, two helpers are essential. They should stand on opposite sides of the bed and take the change of position in stages. The first step is for each helper to place an arm behind the shoulder on his or her side, and together to pull him up and forward. His head should be brought forward, with the chin on the chest.

Once the patient is in the sitting position, the two carers should turn slightly, so that their shoulders nearer the bedhead rest against the back of the patient's shoulder on their side. This lets the carers change their grips, so that they can lift the patient back towards the pillows.

They then move their arm that is resting against the patient's back across his back and down, so that the hand grips the hip bone (or the top of the pyjama trousers) on the other side.

The two carers have now crossed their arms across the patient's back. Then they slip their other arms under the patient's thighs, as near as possible to the buttock, and, with a count to three, lift together, carrying him back to the pillows. When they lift the patient, they should keep up the forward pressure on his shoulders, so that most of his weight is over his knees and not his buttocks.

Many stroke victims can help themselves to sit up. Only one helper is needed. He or she should hold the patient in the same way.

The patient should be' asked to sit well forward, put his unaffected hand flat on the bed, just beside and behind his body, and to bend up his unaffected leg, digging his heel into the mattress. Then, when the carer gives the order 'lift', the patient pushes with heel and hand at the same time as the helper raises him up. The harder the carer presses behind the patient's shoulder, the easier it is to move him.

It is only when the stroke victim tries to sit up in bed that he will fully appreciate the severity of the loss of balance that follows every stroke. He will fall towards his affected side and be wholly unable to maintain even a semi-upright position without support.

It is vital, therefore, that there are enough pillows and cushions to support his weak side, and to keep his arm and leg in the correct positions (elbow and wrist straight, knee and ankle bent). He should not be left alone until it has been made absolutely certain that he will not fall either to the injured side, or worse still, out of bed or his chair.

Four pillows are needed to help him sit. The first two are placed horizontally, one on top of the other. The third is placed vertically behind the patient's affected side, pushing the shoulder blade forwards. He should now be sitting almost bolt upright. The last pillow is now placed behind his head, so that it does not loll to one side, and is not arched backwards.

Once the patient is sitting up and stable, the leg position needs attention. A rolled towel placed from under the buttock to the knee on the affected side keeps both the hip and knee relaxed, preventing muscle contraction. A cradle over the feet takes the pressure of the bedclothes from the ankle joint. Splints are not used to keep joints straight after stroke, as they may weaken the muscles further. The overriding aim is to help the patient to remain aware of his 'lost' limbs and, as soon as possible, to use them.

Stroke victims should not be so propped up that they cannot move. A vital principle of such early care is to encourage the movement, as far as possible, of the paralyzed side of the body. This is not as difficult as it seems. Although after most hemiplegic strokes, patients cannot voluntarily move the limbs on their affected sides, particular movements of the unaffected limbs can encourage automatic stretching and relaxation of the affected paralyzed muscles.

One way to achieve this is to make sure that the patient has to stretch across his affected side with his good arm to reach what he needs. So, although in the early days his tray or bedside table should be placed on his good side, to help correct any slump towards his weak side, it should be changed to the bad side as soon as he becomes used to sitting up and feels stable.

Having to turn his whole body towards his affected side in this way not only helps to keep the affected side of the body from becoming contracted and stiff, it also helps the patient to accept the existence of his 'lost' side. As with turning in bed, however, care must be taken to ensure that the affected arm is not put under abnormal twisting or pressure while the unaffected arm is being used.

*Bed exercises*

Even when lying in bed, patients can exercise their own affected muscles. They should start as soon as they are able to co-operate with their carers, and repeat the exercises several times a day.

The first is for the arms. The bad hand should be gripped by the good one, and the arms lifted over the head, then from side to side. The patient may initially need help to interlace his fingers, and the arm will feel very heavy, but the feeling of achievement will usually compensate for the effort required. It is good for the patient to look at his hands as he does this exercise, as it will help him regain his sense of position. It is not a good idea to use an overhead pulley, as this can pull the shoulder joint out of position.

'Bridging' is an exercise for the trunk, stomach and leg muscles. Lying on his back, with legs bent up so that his feet are flat on the mattress, he should try to lift his buttocks off the bed, then lower them slowly back down. He may need help at first with a hand pressing up behind the small of his back. By doing this, he is putting weight on both feet: the more he can do so, the higher he will raise his buttocks, and the easier it will be to slide a bedpan underneath him.

Swinging the knees from side to side, keeping them together, helps keep the hip and leg muscles in shape. Rolling from side to side, as described above, is also of great benefit, as it not only helps all the torso muscles, but will also prevent bedsores that would otherwise be caused by lying for long periods on one area of skin

*Getting out of bed*

Many patients are well enough to get out of bed within forty-eight hours of their stroke. The first need is to procure the right chair! An armchair with a high seat; a broad seat and a straight back is ideal. The aim is for the patient to be able to sit with his knees at a right angle - thighs horizontal and lower legs vertical, with feet flat on the floor.

The first step is for the patient to roll to the side of the bed, on to his affected side, facing the helper. Both feet should be lifted over the side of the bed. Then the carer should put one hand behind the affected shoulder, and the other around the thighs, as close to the knees as possible. By pushing up on the shoulder blade and forward with the hand around the thigh, the patient should swing up to a sitting position, with legs over the bedside.

He can then be rocked forward, with pressure behind the buttocks, to the edge of the bed. This rocking from side to side is very useful for the patient to learn, as he can use it himself to move around his bed in the sitting position. If he cannot control his sitting position, he can interlace his fingers and hang his arms around the carer's shoulders for support.

Many patients soon learn to help themselves to sit over the side of the bed. Once rolled on to their affected side, with legs bent, they bring their unaffected arm across to the mattress in front of them, and push downwards to lift themselves up, so that they end up, leaning on their affected forearm. They can then push their feet over the side of the bed, and with a further push by the unaffected hand, sit up. Someone should be close by when the patient first attempts this maneuver, as it is easy for them to fail, and fall.

Now that the patient is sitting on the side of the bed, he should practice putting weight on his affected hand and foot. The hands, fingers and thumbs spread out, should be flat on the bed, and the feet flat on the floor. Help will be needed to keep the affected elbow straight. He should then be encouraged to sway from side to side, so that he is putting weight on both arms and legs. A good exercise is to get him to try to resist the pressure of the carer in pushing him, gently from side to side. This has to be done carefully, so that the pressure is smooth and not enough to cause him to over-balance.

*Into a chair*

The crucial points about transfer from bed to chair are that the patient should begin by being as close as possible to the edge of the bed, that his feet are apart and well behind him, and that he should lean forward. The open seat of the chair should be facing the foot of the bed, its side being next to the bedside, alongside the pillows.

He should interlace his fingers and place his arms around his helper's shoulders. The helper then leans forward, bends his knees, puts both hands round the patient's back, low down, and pulls the patient forward over one shoulder. Then as the helper leans back the patient will rise off the bed. The action is more a pulling of the patient forward than of lifting.

With both sets of knees pressed together, it is then possible for the carer to pivot the patient across until his back is facing the chair. He can then sit down on the slow release of the pressure of the two sets of knees. During this movement, he remains leaning forward until he is actually sitting down.

The same movements should be followed when moving the patient back to bed, and from chair to commode. The fronts of the chair and commode should be set at a right angle, the corners touching.

With progress, many patients soon learn to transfer themselves between bed and chair without the need for help. They lean forward to transfer their weight over their feet, placing the unaffected hand beside them on the bed. By pushing down on that hand, they can pivot themselves so that their backs are opposite the chair. They can then lower themselves on to the chair, while still leaning forward. During the turn between bed and chair, all the weight is put on the unaffected side to begin with, but with practice most patients soon learn to share the weight between the two legs. Carers can stand behind patients for the first few attempts to prevent them from falling backwards.

Once in the chair, the leg positions are easy to maintain. If the affected foot rolls on to its outside edge, a thin cushion under the buttock on the same side may help to keep it straight. The arm can be rested on a cushion to keep the shoulders level and the elbow straight, with a pillow behind the affected shoulder blade to stop the shoulder from falling backwards and down. An extra cushion can be used to keep the wrist cocked. The palm of the affected hand can be placed to face the ceiling with the fingers outstretched, or facing downwards on a pillow with the fingers and thumb straight and separated.

It is a mistake to leave the patient grasping any object. This may leave the fingers curled up tightly into a ball, so that if some nerve recovery occurs the fixed contracted muscles cannot respond, even to intense physiotherapy.

Moving a relatively immobile and heavy body around a bed and from a bed to a chair may seem, at first sight, impossible. However, the maneuvers described in this chapter have been designed to reduce the strain on the carer to the minimum. If you follow them closely, you may be surprised how easy they are. It is best, however, to let your professional help - the nurse and physiotherapist – give you a little training in them at first. It also helps to coax your 'patient' into giving a little help - with their good side. The more they can help themselves to move position, the better the long-term outlook - for you too.

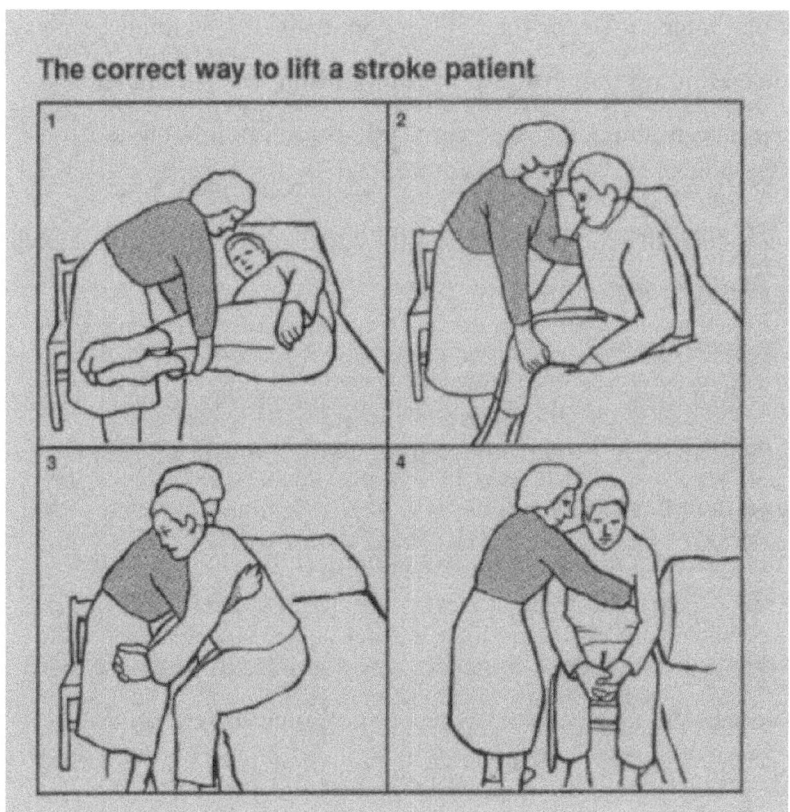

**The correct way to lift a stroke patient**

*Chair exercises*

The hand-clasping exercise described for the bed can be adapted for the chair. The hands are stretched out over a table in front of the chair: the further forward they can be stretched, the better for the trunk muscles and the feet, which should be placed well back.

Raising the hands towards the ceiling comes next: it is much more strenuous. Holding the arms out in front of him, the patient should then swing them to each side in turn. Finally, without a table, he should try to bend over and touch his feet. A refinement of this, which comes with practice, is to run the hands down the shin of each leg in turn towards the ankle.

*Ready to walk again*

The aim of all these exercises is to prepare the patient to walk again. Before that can start, he must be able to sit by himself without leaning to the affected side.

Relearning to walk needs professional help. It takes place in the hospital physiotherapy department, where each person's needs are assessed and the staff have the necessary equipment. They are there, too, to advise the family on how best to continue the exercises at home. Home carers must meet with the hospital staff regularly to discuss how best to continue helping their mutual patient between the hospital visits. The combination of expert help in hospital and enthusiastic application of the expert's advice at home leads to the best possible chance of maximum recovery for the patient.

As movement returns, the occupational therapist in the hospital will be brought in, so that the best practical use can be made of the new-found physical improvement. This step can be a big boost to the morale, especially if the patient can be helped towards regaining a skill that he thought he had lost for good.

The one skill that all stroke patients are desperate to regain is that of easy communication with everyone around them. In the hospital this is the field of the speech therapist, but the main responsibility for bringing the dysphasic patient back into the world of inter-relating human beings must lie with the people who have most contact with him - his family and friends at home. Ways in which this can be done are described in the next chapter.

# 6 Beginning to Live Again

You should challenge the stroke patient or your relatives or friend to come alive again - with humor, with games, with programs to revive old skills.

Be patient, highly inventive, sensitive and practical.

Your philosophy of treating the stroke patient should have three main aspects:

- First, it is the whole person that matters, the spirit, as well as the mind and body.

- Support, effort and humor all help towards the fight for recovery and the acceptance of lingering handicaps.

- Life after a stroke can be lived as fully as possible, despite the handicaps.

Find weekly get-togethers, so that small groups of patients and volunteers meet. Outings and functions are arranged there.

Your task is daunting, because the communication problems left by a stroke are complex. It is not just a matter of being unable to speak.

Questions that must be answered include:

- Can he understand others speaking to him?

- Can he read?

- If he can read, can he remember what he read a few minutes ago?

- Can he write? Does he recognize shapes, like letters?

- If he was right handed, can he now write with his left?

- How is he with numbers, or the time, or money?

- Can he plan ahead, or initiate an action?

The lack of communication does not mean that all intellect is lost. The stroke victim has not become a child again: he is bewildered, frustrated and depressed by his predicament. There is even a real sense of grief at what the stroke has taken away from him. The resulting low morale and lack of self-confidence may well lead to a downward drift into apathy, despair and indifference to the help of others or to the future.

So helping stroke victims is more than just improving the mechanics of communication. They need company throughout the day: they need to be entertained, to have their spirits raised, to be given hope for a future in which they are better than they are now.

Somehow, their helpers must instil into them a sense of purpose and self respect, and at the same time steer them away from selfishness, cynicism and apathy.

They must work towards their own recovery and expect no miracle cure. Many must be helped to come to terms with residual disabilities, often along with the realization that their plans for the future - in a career, sport or travel, for example - may have to be drastically revised.

For the Stroke Volunteers, the way towards recovery is based on two main themes - interest and stimulation. Helpers - and many patients do best with a team, each member of which will visit for a short time on a regular basis - need to know how to gain the patient's interest. Everything depends on his interests before the stroke. As the writers of *A Time to Speak* point out, it is no use giving a football fanatic a copy of *Woman's Own* to read: far better to give him the report of yesterday's match.

In the same vein, the racing fan can be given the day's race card and coaxed into acting as the family bookmaker for the day - organizing betting odds and picking favorites. Housewives who have been used to cooking for a family could be challenged to plan and prepare a meal - of course with the aid of a carer commis-chef. It is amazing what can be done with only one good arm, even in a kitchen.

The key to improvement is a lively atmosphere around the patient. Along with stimulating interest comes laughter and friendship. The relationship between carer and patient should be much more like that between equal friends than of teacher and pupil. It is not a bad thing for the carer to make the odd mistake and to be put right by the patient: when a stroke patient wins a game of draughts or cards it can be a big boost to his morale.

Even in the best-run households, however, there are long periods when the patient is left on his own. This is more difficult for him than many people realize, because the normal train of thought and imagination may be disturbed, leaving him in a form of mental limbo which can be very unpleasant. This means that helpers must plan for him the periods in which he is alone, so that he can be kept occupied, as much as possible. Most of us wake every morning knowing that we have set tasks ahead of us that we must complete.

The stroke victim has lost this privilege: he does not know how to organize his day or what he has to do. Much of the time ahead he sees as a void that he has no way of filling: it is up to the carers to do that for him.

One way to do this is to organize a series of visitors – neighbors and friends - who will arrive at different times and bring different tasks and interests with them. An open desk diary for everyone to use acts as a mental aide in a series of ways: it is a reminder of past events, as well as of what the days and weeks ahead hold, from the day's television program to a future holiday or family birthday.

The diary also shows up empty days that might be better filled by visiting friends or volunteers. The patient can be encouraged to use it as a personal diary, noting who came and what they did together. Visitors can use it to leave messages for one another. All these purposes lead to added interest for the patient - an excellent treatment aid for the expense only of a diary and a pen.

Days that appear empty can be filled by activities that we all take for granted, but that for the stroke victim are a challenge that has to be met. He should be encouraged, for example, to share in the household chores, such as dusting, table laying, and putting away the cutlery. Cooking and gardening can be organized with only one hand, as can looking after houseplants or feeding the pet. An aquarium or a pet budgerigar can give hours of interest and pleasure. Although activity through the day rather than rest should be a priority, it is good to set aside a particular time of day for a rest. Planning it to coincide with a radio or television program helps to avoid boredom or introspection. Schools' and children's television programs can be surprisingly interesting and educational for an adult stroke victim. Indoor games such as jigsaws and patience are also interest raisers, but it is good to get outside at least once a day.

Staying indoors for days on end, no matter how well the days are filled, can be depressing and restraining.

Once all this enthusiasm for helping the patient has started, it is common to forget another important person - the patient's spouse or closest relative, usually a daughter, who has to bear the main burden. This person must be able to get away from the burden without feeling guilty or ashamed. He or she has his or her own life to lead and must be able to do so, otherwise the burden will become too much to bear. In any case, the patient benefits from hearing about life outside the home, which can easily turn into a prison for both patient and carer if some time off is not arranged. In these circumstances, resentment can easily build up on both sides and relationships, however happy previously, can break down.

This is where a good band of friends and volunteers is invaluable. They provide interest, variety and support, and a safety valve for the main carer. Without them it is difficult, if not impossible, for the carer to struggle on alone.

# 7 Learning Language Again

As mentioned earlier, the worst aspect of a stroke for many people is not the paralysis, but the loss of language. Whether this is dysphasia, when damage to the brain has made it difficult to 'think of the right word' or dysarthria (in which there are no problems in being able to understand speech, but the muscles controlling the actual production of sound in the larynx have been affected by the stroke), the distress is always severe, and the defect needs urgent attention from the very first days after the stroke.

Language problems after a stroke cannot always be corrected, but there is almost always a way to improve them. This is not just the responsibility of the professional speech therapist: family and friends have much to offer in retraining the dysphasic or dysarthric patient. However, the speech therapist does have the first task: a detailed assessment of the type and severity of the language deficit. Speech therapists today are highly expert in the analysis of language problems and in how to correct them. Every doctor who has had to deal with stroke patients would agree that they can perform miracles, provided they have enough time with their patients.

However, as is the case with so many medical services, there are far too few speech therapists for the number of people, not only stroke patients, who need their attention. The next best option is for the closest carers to be briefed by the therapist on what must be done that will best help their particular patient. The speech and language management will then be carried out at home, with regular visits to the therapist to assess progress and draw up further plans.

This scheme often works very well, but some carers have to face up to the realization that their stroke victim will never fully recover all his powers of language. In such cases, substitutes, such as sign language, printed messages and even abstract symbols may be helpful.

Early predictions of how much speech will be recovered are not always dependable. Some people given pessimistic outlooks for recovery of speech do remarkably well, even after many months of apparent hopelessness. Perseverance and unflagging optimism are always preferable to, and often much more realistic than, pessimism. Recovery of speech is gradual and often takes months. Progress is usually stepwise, so that there are sometimes weeks with no change, followed by a day in which a sudden improvement takes everyone, including the patient, by a pleasant surprise. Dysphasia, more than dysarthria perhaps, causes the most anxiety and difficulty between patient and carers. Happily, it is the language problem that is most likely to improve and even disappear, especially with intensive encouragement from friends. So the message is to keep at it, even if there is no immediate progress.

Speech retraining can take several forms. One is 'melodic intonation therapy', or MIT. Many dysphasic patients can sing words that they cannot speak, apparently because musical skills are controlled by one half of the brain, and speech by the other. In MIT the speech therapist first sings a short sentence, then asks the patient to copy it. With success, the short sentences become longer and more intricate. Patients do not have to be musical to be successful!

Speech therapists combine a tapped out rhythm with MIT, so that the patient can use the rhythm himself - say, by tapping with a pencil to strict timing - to help make the process of speech more automatic. When the mind is on one thing, it is easier to accomplish the other. If the patient can get the hang of the singing and tapping early, they can both be gradually diminished, leaving normal speech in their place.

Most dysphasics who benefit from MIT and rhythm therapy have retained their comprehension of speech, but have problems in expressing themselves. Those who have lost understanding of speech may need a different approach.

One way to help them is to read out what one wants to say from a book or a printed text, pointing to the words on the page at the same time as they are pronounced. It is best to stick to meaningful sentences when doing this, and not to concentrate on single words.

An added approach is to use sign language. One in particular, Amerind, adapted from the language of North American Indians, is simpler than most, easier to use and understand, and most importantly is possible using one hand. Naturally, the carers have to learn it as well as the stroke victim. It has not found much favor on the Eastern side of the Atlantic, but can be very useful for patients with profound and persistent speech defects who obviously retain their understanding of language.

This recognition of sign language as a method of communication has led some therapists to translate this to the printed page. For a few patients who cannot recognize the alphabet, symbols to replace words and ideas have been used instead with success. They can be made up onto plastic cards and used to communicate everyday messages between carer and patient.

There is also a strong case for group therapy in speech training. New stroke patients who have communication difficulties often find a one-to-one meeting with the doctor or the speech therapist quite daunting. When other stroke patients are included, the patients can learn from each other and quickly come to realize that they are not the only people in the world with such difficulties. A camaraderie builds up in the group that can both raise the mood and speed up the process of learning. Several patients can benefit from the results of one person's efforts, whether they are successes or mistakes. In particular, learning in a group helps people to lose their fear that they will make fools of themselves - something that would otherwise greatly hinder their progress.

*Working with words*

Although the speech therapist will start the process of recovering the ability to communicate, the main burden falls on the family and friends at home, who are often at a loss about what to do. Among the ways they can offer practical help are the following:

- Don't try to force words out of patients. They will come naturally in conversation, especially when the context is humor, or when the subject is of particular interest to the patient.

- Always speak clearly, slightly slower than usual, and pause at the appropriate grammatical moments, such as at the end of a phrase or a sentence.

- Be careful not to drop your voice at the end of a sentence: this is a common fault that can confuse even the keenest of listeners.

On the other hand, *never* shout: strokes do not make people deaf, and shouting at a stroke patient smacks of condescension.

- Sit opposite the patient as you speak, so that he can see your lips and facial expression. Both can help to convey the sense of what you say, along with the words.

- Do speak a lot! The more the patient is stimulated, the more likely he is to recover more quickly.

- Give him lots of time to respond, but also be prepared to help, by prompting, if he is in obvious difficulty.

- Use word puzzles to increase interest and vocabulary

- Ask questions (to which you know the answer!) to try to elicit a response and stimulate logical thought. The 'Twenty Questions' format, in which the patient needs only to answer 'yes' or 'no', is ideal to begin with.

- Ask patients to name objects put into their hands: this helps to link language with shape and space.
- Ask them to name everyday things around them, such as the furniture or crockery, and add questions about their shape, color or number.
- Don't hesitate to repeat exercises: this helps the memory, and as the patient improves with practice, he will feel a sense of achievement.
- Go outdoors and do the same for objects in the garden, or seen on a journey.
- Sit by a window and watch the world around you: this gives more scope for interest and helps to bring the patient out of himself. The patient's chair should face a window, rather than the wall opposite.
- Choose a subject that you know interests the patient, and buy books and magazines on it. It is amazing how conversation can be built up around the advertising, as well as the main articles. If there are illustrations to the text, so much the better. Comic papers can be a great help in linking words to pictures.
- Help to compile an old-fashioned scrap book about a subject dear to the patient. This can be left with him at times when he is alone, to organize and plan, and to mull over.

- Hark back to the most important past experiences. Many people look back on the war as the most meaningful time in their lives, when they made their greatest contribution to society. Usually; the younger generation people react to such reminiscences with 'Oh, no, not again'. This is the time to encourage them, as remembering these times can be a powerful stimulus to other· memories. Once memory starts to return, the flood gates sometimes open, and improvement in memory and understanding can be speedy and surprisingly complete.

- Bring out maps and postcards of familiar places, and try to stimulate anecdotes of what happened where. Even street maps can be a source of surprising interest.

- Old family photographs are often a winner, whether the carer is a relative or not. Explaining to an outsider who all these people are, and who were the black sheep or the odd ones out, can often lead to laughter and happy memories - as can reminiscing about them with the people who knew them. Old memories like these can elicit powerful reactions and emotions that would not be stirred by any other subject.

All these stimuli must contribute towards improvement in understanding and memory, which may well lead to the bonus of improved speech.

Even when speech remains very difficult, sharing non-verbal games and occupations, such as jigsaws or painting, can remove the patient's stress at trying to talk. Under such circumstances, carer and patient may find themselves exchanging words almost without knowing it. Sometimes taking the mind off the problem for a while can help to overcome it.

Once speech starts to return, the classical old parlor games on words can offer real scope for improvement in language skills.

Besides 'Twenty Questions', I-spy, charades, animal vegetable and mineral, consequences and board games such as 'Scrabble' can be a real stimulus for the patient and something that the whole family can enjoy. Scrabble letters can also be used to make up favorite word games, such as anagrams.

The relaxed atmosphere while playing such games can bring grandchildren and an affected grandparent, for example, much closer. Feeling in tune with all the generations in the family can ease the patient's state of mind - and a teenager interested in helping a much-loved grandparent through the early days of a stroke can be a marvelous boost to the old man's or old woman's morale.

The list of ways in which the ability of the patient to understand and use words is virtually endless. Quizzes, picture puzzles, searching for names in atlases, word association games, crosswords and even secret messages and simple codes can keep up interest.

Carers wishing to know more should refer to *A Time to Speak,* in which there are detailed instructions for several word games and exercises specifically designed to help the stroke sufferer.

*Reading again*

Reading is a skill that many people, not themselves keen readers, take for granted until they lose it. Only then do they understand the problems in not being able to read destinations on buses, or labels on goods for sale, or instructions for appliances, or radio or television programs - or a host of other everyday essentials. And these problems fade into insignificance for the person who, before his stroke, loved reading and can no longer recognize the printed word. For many stroke victims an apparent reading problem has its roots in poor vision or poor speech. They can read if the print is large, in the best light, and the book is placed within the half of the field of vision that remains. They may not be able to read aloud because their speech is impaired but, left with a book, they can enjoy reading quietly to themselves. Many, too, have a short concentration, so that they can only enjoy reading and retain what they have read if they stop after a few minutes.

Others have poor short-term memory, so that they quickly forget what they have read only a few minutes before. Unless this improves, reading - and most other activities - is meaningless to them.

Rules about reading for a stroke victim include:

- choose clear, well-spaced large print (large print books are available from libraries);

- choose good light and make use of reading glasses (reading glasses and special aids such as line by line readers can be obtained through the hospital and local ophthalmic opticians);

- cover the line below, and possibly the line above, the one being read, so that the eye is helped to keep on the same line;

- the carer should read with the patient using another copy of the same book, to help in prompting;
- carer and patient should read aloud together at times, with the patient just following the carer;
- question the patient afterwards, on what he has read: this gives a good idea of his level of understanding;
- get him to read a newspaper every day. Even if he can only read the headlines, this is helpful, and can lead not just to improvement in reading ability, but to interest in the outside world.

For a rest from reading, members of the family should take it in turns to read aloud to the patient. Those living away from home can send in tapes of their news. Libraries now loan taped books, so that the patient can read and listen to the same words simultaneously. For some patients this not only improves their enjoyment of life, it also rapidly improves their reading and understanding skills. It gives the rest of the family a break and the patient something to organize for himself when alone.

*Writing*

If speech is impaired, then the ability to write becomes very important. It is not only that signatures are needed for pension books and cheques: sometimes the only way that a patient with apraxia (mechanical speech problem) can communicate is by writing notes and passing them round. Of course, if the stroke-affected hand is the one with which the patient learned to write, then the patient may have a double difficulty - his stroke-induced problem with language, and the clumsiness of the remaining unaffected hand. Many stroke victims resist, at first, the idea of changing their writing hand. Most, however, co-operate when they begin to understand how important the need to write has become, even if the writing itself is far below their usual standard.

It is important to give the would-be writer every chance of success. He cannot hold down the paper with his other hand, so it must be fixed: a clipboard is one good answer. An elastic band wound round the shaft of a pen or pencil gives a better grip.

Nowadays, however, many households have microcomputers and word processors. Learning to use the keyboard is both satisfying and an excellent self-improvement aid. Using the computer, for creative writing, correspondence, and even computer games, can give endless enjoyment to patients who must spend hours alone each day. The games, indeed, can sharpen reactions, and many hospital rehabilitation units now use them to help patients with special problems. They can be used just as easily and just as effectively in the home.

# 8 Everyday Problems: memory, concentration, number, time, money

Because strokes leave people paralyzed and unable to speak, their other problems are apt to be underestimated and even neglected. Yet they have a series of other problems that interfere with the everyday activities that the rest of us take for granted. If they are neglected it is difficult, if not impossible, for them to return to an independent lifestyle.

Think, for a moment, of how you could manage if: your memory for recent events was so poor that you could not remember what happened this morning; your ability to concentrate on any subject lasted only a few minutes; you found it hard to organize and remember otherwise familiar shapes and objects; you could no longer add up simple numbers, did not know the value of money could no longer tell the time and your color sense had gone.

This is the state in which many stroke patients find themselves. It would be difficult enough if they also had full movement of all their limbs and complete control over their speech: when paralysis and aphasia are added, the problems seem insurmountable.

Yet there are ways to help people climb back, provided their carers know what to do. The hospital occupational and speech therapists will help all they can to put patients on the right lines but, as with difficulties in movement and in communications, most of the work must be done in the home by those closest to them.

*Memory*

Most stroke patients retain their memory for the distant past. Childhood memories can be particularly clear, but what has happened only a few minutes before is forgotten. This does not mean that they are living in the past: they would love to remember the present, but need considerable help to be able to do so.

Carers, therefore, have constantly to jog the patient's memory about what is happening throughout the day. In the morning, with the diary to hand, they should talk through yesterday's activities and make plans for the day to come. Constant repetition of what needs to be remembered helps to improve memory, even in a brain damaged by a stroke.

Words and pictures are remembered in different ways by the brain, so that tests of both should be set, repeatedly and preferably in a light-hearted atmosphere. Games that use short-term memory abound. In Pelmanism, each player is asked in turn to choose two cards from a pack spread haphazardly, face down on a table. The aim is to pick pairs of numbers. The winner is usually the one who best remembers the cards that his opponents turn up.

Another is a 'list' game. It starts with the first player saying 'I went to market, and bought ... '. He or she mentions one purchase.

The second player must repeat the first purchase and add a second.

The third has then to list three purchases, and the game continues until someone makes a mistake. Most people will know several variants of this type of game.

Card or board games, like whist or chess, are also useful stimulants of short-term memory. It does not matter if the patient played them before the stroke or not, as the discipline of taking in a new set of rules helps to develop memory and logical thought. They have the advantage of being played with partners or opponents, who can help when the patient makes mistakes or gets into trouble, or even panics. Computer games are more solitary but they can help to stimulate memory, provided they are very 'user friendly', and there are people nearby who can provide guidance.

Visual memory can be stimulated by the old parlor game in which the patient is asked to stare at a picture for a fixed number of minutes, then asked questions about its contents. Something similar can be done with a tray filled with household objects: after it has been examined, two objects are removed and the patient asked to look again to identify the missing pieces.

All these games aim to train the brain to renew systems of memory that have been lost in the stroke. They are best undertaken in a spirit of relaxation and humor, and not as exercises almost similar to school room tests. When the patient becomes tired, stop for a while and turn to something else, but it is important to organize some time, every day, for memory stimulation. Not everyone responds, but when people do the result can be very rewarding.

*Concentration*

Stroke patients quickly tire. Their concentration span for anyone subject or occupation can be as short as a few minutes. When their enthusiasm is obviously flagging, it is time to transfer to another occupation or activity: it is easier for them to start concentrating again on a different subject than to continue. However, gentle but firm persuasion can help to extend the concentration span, so that over weeks it can be doubled or more. The more interesting a subject is to the patient, the longer he will concentrate on it, so carers who are really successful are usually enthusiasts themselves!

One way to kindle interest and to improve concentration is to take the patient out of his environment. Remember that most stroke patients are imprisoned behind the four walls of their home. It is usually a safe, comfortable, familiar environment, the one that is best for maximal recovery, but it can be boring. Boredom breeds inactivity and that, in turn, worsens the ability to concentrate. An outing with friends immediately increases awareness of the outside world, and with that comes heightened powers of observation and concentration.

*Number skills*

The stroke victim's loss of recognition of letters and words often obscures the fact that he has also become less numerate. Yet numbers play almost as big a part as letters in our lives, from the numbers on our door, clocks, phones and calendars to those in our accounts and bank statements.

Stroke patients can find even the simplest of numbers too much, and for some they remain so. However, many can be trained at least to cope with the numbers they must deal with in day-to-day life - such as shopping, travel tickets, dialing on the telephone, changing small sums of money, and even taking an interest in the household accounts.

Fortunately there are many aids to improving number skills. Number puzzle books abound, and card and dice games depend on knowing and adding numbers. Children's games such as ludo and bagatelle (or pinball) can be enjoyed as much by grandparents as by their grandchildren - and even more so when they play together. Among other useful games for relearning number skills are backgammon, bingo, roulette and darts.

Probably most important of all, however, for developing social as well as number skills, are the various card games with scoring systems that rely on simple addition and memory. Among them are whist, gin rummy, pontoon, poker and bridge. Cribbage is an excellent test of arithmetic for two people, and patience for one. Dominoes, too, help both to improve numeric skills and to re-establish social skills among people with strokes. Those whose number skills have improved faster than their word skills feel comfortable when they meet old friends over a game of dominoes. Their natural shyness diminishes as the players have to concentrate on the numbers - and the differences between them become less marked.

*Time*

A specific problem with numbers is inability to tell the time. If the ability to understand the 24-hour clock has been lost, patients can easily become disorientated: night can be turned into day, with all that this means in disturbance to the family.

However, most problems with telling the time are just that – the patient cannot communicate with others about the time, but in fact is still in touch with the time of day and the daily routine.

Nevertheless, it should be made as easy as possible for him to know the time and to be able to communicate about it to others. To do this, he needs a watch or clock with the traditional round face, and the usual arithmetical, rather than Roman, numerals. Sometimes the two hands are confusing: a watchmaker can take off the minute hand and leave a perfectly useful watch which can be read with an accuracy of around two minutes.

There are many teaching aids, such as large clock faces with movable hands, for children to learn to tell the time: most stroke patients are not in the least insulted if they are asked to work with one.

As skills with understanding time improve, the training can move on to include bus and railway timetables. If he has been a driver, the patient has drastic changes to make in his life, one of which may well be that he has to use public transport from now on.

Understanding calendars is also important, not just so that the patient knows the day of the week and the month, but also that he knows when family birthdays are due. The simple act of remembering a birthday can be a boost to confidence: finding afterwards that he has forgotten one can badly dent a patient's self-esteem.

*Money*

One of the biggest mistakes people make when caring for stroke patients is to take over the management of all their money. Obviously, many spouses or sons or daughters must take over the general responsibility for household money management from their stroke-afflicted relative. However, dignity demands that the patient is left with some money to use on his own behalf. People feel left out, understandably, if they cannot offer to pay for a drink or buy sweets for a grandchild. Without money, they have no means of returning to any semblance of normal living.

So, after a stroke, patients who are mobile should be helped first to plan, then to go on, shopping expeditions, not just for everyday things but to buy presents for family and friends - perhaps as a token of gratitude for help over the bad period, or as birthday or Christmas gifts.

The feeling of being in control of one's own decisions is very important to rehabilitation, and nowhere more so than in being able to spend one's money the way one wishes. However, this is an area that often needs close supervision. The simple problem of counting numbers is complicated by difficulties in differentiating between the various coins and banknotes - even the feel of the coins may now be strange. Mistakes can be made that would be regretted later if not checked before the money is handed over.

Because of this, it is good to practice shopping at home, using real money, before going out for the first time. It is also a good idea to choose, for that first outing, a shop that clearly displays price tickets on all their goods, so that the money to be paid can be organized in time before it has to be paid.

Asking the patient to check the bill in a restaurant is another good training exercise - it is amazing how often some bills are wrong, and how good the patient will feel if he spots a mistake!

*Manipulating shapes*

Problems with recognizing shapes and in appreciating perspective are difficult to assess in stroke patients. If the vision has been affected, as in most hemiplegic patients, it can be assumed that there are difficulties in recognizing objects and in judging where they are in space.

As patients improve this facility is relearned, but relatively slowly. One way to help improve the progress is to set up a jigsaw. Jigsaws are very good training aids for improving perception of color and shape, and for developing manipulative skills in the fingers and hand. They are also excellent pastimes for whiling away the odd hour between visitors. They range widely in their complexity, so that one can always be chosen to suit a particular patient's needs and interests.

Another 'shape' game to improve perceptive skills is the Tangram, a set of cut-out cardboard shapes that can be put together in all sorts of different ways to produce elegant designs and figures.

Apparently an ancient Chinese game, its interest has been proved over several thousand years and patients with no verbal skills can become quite proficient at it.

*Organizing stroke support*

You will have recognized by now that families, friends and volunteers can be crucial to the extent to which a stroke victim can recover. However, no matter how enthusiastic and energetic the carers are, they need professional help to organize and plan the way ahead.

The hospital staff of physician, physiotherapist, speech therapist and occupational therapist will liaise with the home care team of the family doctor, district and nurses, physiotherapist, and social worker to help the patient and his family.

They do this by providing *people,* almost all of whom have gone through the same trauma and who understand. They offer tangible relief, and practical solutions to the immediate problems. They can make the crucial difference to home care, so that the patient who would otherwise have to stay in a permanent nursing home or hospital care may be able to stay at home.

# 9 Stroke and Sexuality

As long ago as 1974 a British survey of the sexual problems of disabled people revealed that half of them had sexual problems so severe that they were very unhappy. The more severe their physical disability, the more difficult it was for them to achieve sexual satisfaction. However, at the root of most of the problems was not the physical handicap, but the prevailing psychological attitudes towards sex among the disabled and their partners. Physical decline was equated wrongly with sexual decline, so that the thought that disabled people could be interested, or even indulge, in sexual activity was discouraged, ignored by or even abhorrent to many people.

This was nothing short of a tragedy for many stroke victims. Sexuality does not decline with age. It changes, so that there is perhaps less emphasis on the physical side of the sex act itself, but there is still a powerful need, even when we are old, to be close to someone of the opposite sex and to feel wanted. The attraction between older men and women is more subtle than that between young adults, but it is definitely there and needs to be expressed physically as well as emotionally.

The belief that sexual activity tends to stop as we pass middle age has no basis in fact. Many older women find the menopause a great release from periods and the fear of pregnancy, and find that they can enjoy sex more than ever before. Claims that men lose their potency as they age are also exaggerated. The lower sexual activity of older men is probably due more to lessening opportunity than to declining sexual ability. And even if the physical side of sex has declined so that erections are slower to arise, shorter in duration and less complete, the interest in sex remains.

The truth is, no matter what is said or believed in public, most happily married couples continue their active sex lives well into advanced old age. They may not admit it to others, but they continue to enjoy sex as an expression of their love for one another and for the pleasure that it gives both of them.

For men or women who have enjoyed a full sex life before a stroke, its complete loss afterwards can be a disaster just as severe to them as aphasia or paralysis. The problem, however, is that its effect on the psyche is hidden. Many older patients feel that they must conform to the accepted view of their generation that sexuality is something not to be mentioned in decent conversation. They may feel embarrassed to admit that they have even had a recent sex life, thinking that society would disapprove of such behavior at their age!

So their misery may have to be brought into the open, either by the doctor or by one of the professional team in hospital or the district. Obviously, opening the subject to discussion has to be done with tact, dignity and no little courage. Usually, however, the response by the couple is one of immense relief. The doctor often discovers that patients have withdrawn from initiating sexual activity because they feel their disability must have destroyed their partner's feelings of sexual attraction towards them. Their partners, far from losing their feelings for them, have usually shied away from sex because they feel that it may promote another stroke, or make them ill in some other way. Both attitudes add to the couple's misery and deepen the patients' natural depressive response to their physical state.

Once these attitudes have been abandoned most couples can be helped towards enjoying a fulfilling sexual, as well as personal, relationship again. The difference in a couple who have started to share again all that they used to share in marriage before the stroke can be startling. It is often the start of considerable improvement, all round, in the patient's general health and ability to communicate.

Of course, it must be admitted that some strokes have a profound effect on sexuality. The depression that accompanies most strokes also depresses sexual desire, and can deepen further the patient's belief that the stroke has made him less attractive.

There may also be fear that any excitement, including sexual excitement, will provoke another stroke. This risk is very small, but it can be reduced even further by taking sex slowly and calmly, and leaving most of the energetic activity to the healthy partner. The idea that orgasm is necessary for completely satisfactory sex is one that most older couples already recognize as false, but there is no harm and much pleasure in concentrating on bringing one's partner to orgasm while controlling one's own.

Some strokes directly damage the sexual response. Sensation in the sexual organs can be reduced on the side of the stroke, so that the physical satisfaction of sex is reduced. However, if the partner concentrates on stroking and caressing the side that is still sensitive, the response can be as full as ever. It is best to avoid caressing the numb side of the body in people with hemiparesis: since they cannot feel what is being done, it can produce confusion and spoil the intimacy of the moment.

Even paralysis of one side is no real hindrance to a sensitive, loving and caring partnership. The active partner can devise ways of moving and embracing that give mutual pleasure. They do not need to involve full sexual intercourse: mutual genital caressing and oral sex may be just as satisfying, provided that both partners find them wholly acceptable and pleasurable.

Probably the most serious sexual problem after a stroke for men is impotence. In fact, permanent impotence after a stroke is rare, except in those severe cases where there is also incontinence due to loss of the nerve control of bladder and bowel.

Most male stroke patients, therefore, retain their ability to erect. It may be reduced by drugs prescribed after the stroke, for example for high blood pressure, or by tranquillizers, anti-cancer drugs, drugs for Parkinson's disease, and some anti-depressant drugs. Diabetes, especially if it has not been rigidly controlled, may also be linked with impotence. In all these cases, changes in the medical management may well improve things.

In most cases of impotence, however, the underlying cause is psychological. If a patient wakes with a morning erection, there is nothing wrong with the nerve supply to the penis. What is needed is a partner's loving attention, with everything that means in touching, holding, caressing and tenderness. The whole body - at least all the area of skin that still has normal sensation - can be used as an erogenous zone for the partner to stimulate, leaving the penis to last, and most important. Such sexual play must be mutual: the most powerful stimulant to sexual feelings is to find that your partner is sexually aroused. As these feelings arise, and anxiety and depression are allayed, many men will find that their impotence disappears.

For women stroke victims a major problem can be a feeling of loss of femininity, and of being no longer attractive to their partners. Much then depends on the partners' attitude. They must be understanding, tender and loving, and take care to learn all the ways in which they can still give the pleasure that both need. Stroke rarely removes all sensation from the clitoris, so that there is no real equivalent in women to impotence in men. Mutual erogenous caressing can still be as fulfilling for a woman stroke partner as for a man.

Sadly, for some couples, the stroke does cause too many problems for sexual activity to be resumed. The partner may have been too badly damaged for the personality and intellect to re-emerge. The personality that does emerge after the stroke may differ so much - sometimes in an unpleasant direction - from the previous one that the partner's feelings change. The patient's sexual drive may even increase, not necessarily in an acceptable way, so that the partner is repelled by his advances. This last problem, though thankfully rare, needs very special medical advice and care, and spouses should not try to deal with it alone.

However, it would be wrong to end this chapter on a negative note. By far the majority of couples who have endured the catastrophe of a stroke in one partner find that they can resume their sexual partnership, happily and with fulfillment. If those who find that they have sexual problems can overcome their understandable shyness and embarrassment and seek advice, they may well be astonished at how happy they can be even under their new circumstances.

# 10 Mechanical and Other Aids

Think of all the tasks around the home that need two hands, then try to perform them with one. Like cutting a slice of bread or opening a tin, slicing off the top of a boiled egg or undressing for the toilet. Now you can begin to understand just how difficult life is after a stroke.

The basis of most problems is the need to be able to steady things with one hand so that the other can be used to perform the task. If one hand is paralyzed this fixing ability has been lost and the task cannot even be started, far less completed.

Happily" many mechanical and electronic aids for the disabled - details about where they can be obtained will be given by your local branch of The Stroke Association - are ideal for most stroke victims. Although the first principle of rehabilitation is to help patients make the best of their residual abilities, using such aids to make life easier does not hinder progress, and can greatly boost their morale. The more they can do for themselves, and the less they feel a burden to others, the better their quality of life and their outlook for even more improvement.

The two most important areas are the kitchen and bathroom. Most kitchen aids can be fixed to the wall or work surface, so that the fixture removes the need for a steadying hand. Tin openers and gadgets for unscrewing bottle tops and jars can be fixed to the wall. Cordless electric carving knives, kettles and irons avoid the need for constant plugging and unplugging into wall sockets. Special vices can be used to clamp materials to kitchen tables and worktops.

Applying spread to bread slices is easier on boards with raised edges: knives that work on a rocking movement, rather than by sawing, are easier to use if you are one handed. Guards around the edges of plates stop their contents being spilled. Suction cups under plates, saucers and bowls, and magnets under saucepans, stop them moving around on table, worktop or oven. Nails knocked through boards can be used as 'spikes' for vegetables and fruit to make them easier to peel.

Levers can be attached to taps, door handles and keys, and handles can even be stuck on electric plugs. Egg cups have been designed to make it easier to lift boiled eggs from the pot, place them on the plate and steady them for slicing.

In the bathroom, handles fixed to the walls wherever the patient needs to change position, say next to the toilet seat or above the bath, are essential to prevent overbalancing. A board that fits, without budging an inch, in the bottom of the bath makes it easier to climb into and out of the bath. Bath and shower taps should either be close at hand, or fitted with flexible hoses so that the patient can wash all over more easily. Slippery bath mats should be banned from any bathroom, especially one used by a stroke victim whose balance is already suspect.

Most appreciated of all are the systems that allow patients to use the toilet in privacy. Although they are expensive, automatic toilets that wash and blow-dry the anal area are a real boon, and the outlay should be a prime priority for the family. Commodes, too, although always second-best to the use of the normal household toilet, have greatly improved in design, ease of use and hygiene. Today's portable commodes both kill germs and remove the odor.

Incontinence is, naturally, often the most distressing after-effect of stroke for the patient who, even if badly brain damaged, usually still retains his or her sense of shame and embarrassment at the mess that the family must deal with.

Managing bowel and bladder leakages cannot be left to the carer alone. Visiting nurses will advise on the best ways to tackle them, from incontinence pads and sheets to catheters and even surgery. One problem is disposal of wet or soiled waste: this can usually be arranged through the local nursing and social services. Many areas employ specific continence advisers, who should be able to ensure that the patient remains dry and clean.

Armchair design has been ingeniously adapted for stroke patients. Chairs for the disabled have firm back, arm and side supports, with mechanical or electronically-operated systems for raising and tilting that help people to sit and stand with the minimum of effort. Some allow the sitter to adjust himself into a lying position with feet up, not unlike the modem dentist's operating chair or a first-class seat in an intercontinental plane. Lap tables are fully adjustable: some, with loose foam filling, mold themselves across the knees, yet provide a firm surface on which to eat, read or work.

There are even systems for helping people with paralyzed hand but some movement in the upper arm to make as much practical use of the affected arm as possible. Supports can be fitted under the forearm that have at their end a grip for a pen or paintbrush. The patient can then use what shoulder movement he has left to teach himself to paint or draw. Some find similar benefit from systems using an over arm frame with pulleys and springs to hold the forearm in place.

The modem telephones with press-button dialing, memories for regularly used numbers and redialing facilities are also a boon for those who find numbers difficult. Office-type telephones that can be used without the need to lift the receiver are also greatly appreciated, as are cordless phones that can be used within fifty meters of the base. Alarm systems that automatically dial an emergency service simply by pulling on a pen or locket device are another essential for any stroke victim who must spend hours alone. Most cities and towns in Britain have such services for their disabled population. Carers for people with walking difficulties should not rush into buying mobility aids, such as tripods and quadripods, zimmers, crutches and wheelchairs, without waiting to make sure first that they will be needed. Patients who can do without them should be encouraged to manage by themselves as much as they can. There is no doubt, however, that a wheelchair that an enthusiastic but tired would-be walker can collapse into after an hour or two of hard effort can be a good buy.

If buying a wheelchair is being considered, follow the advice of your professional helpers on the type needed for your particular patient. Indoor and outdoor wheelchairs differ considerably in their specifications, and you must be certain which one is needed before making your decision. Once bought, it must be very scrupulously maintained. Badly cared-for tires and brakes can be very dangerous: the wheelchair needs as much regular care as any bicycle.

The classical walking aid is the 'zimmer', a broad frame with four legs, inside which the patient tries to steady himself and shuffle along. Shuffle is the correct description, as zimmers restrict speed and foot movement. The decision to use one should be left to the physiotherapist in charge of the case, and only when there is no other way to promote mobility. This must be relatively rare for most people recovering from stroke.

Much better than the zimmer are elbow crutches, used on both arms, so that the patient begins with the stability of four points of contact, three of them being in touch with the ground at anyone time. As balance and weight bearing improve, the graduation is to a 'three-point' system involving putting the weight on the normal leg, then swinging the two crutches together. The weight is then put on the crutches, while the sound foot is swung forward. This should lead towards 'two-point' walking, in which right leg and left crutch, then left leg and right crutch, take the weight.

Tripods and quadripods are essentially walking sticks with small feet, either three or four, at their bases. People with poor balance find them useful, although it must be said that quadripods are much more stable and are to be preferred to the three-footed support.

A normal walking stick with a good rubber foot and a grip that the patient feels fits his hand is probably the most effective aid for patients who have less severe mobility problems. The length is crucial: when his weight is put upon it, the patient should be standing upright, the elbow slightly bent, and with no hint of a lean to the side or a forward stoop. It should be held in the unaffected hand, and be allowed to swing forward with the opposite foot.

To begin with, most, if not all, the weight of that side of the body will be taken by the stick. As confidence grows, along with better balance, more and more weight will be placed on the affected side. The aim is eventually to discard the stick altogether - unless the patient wishes to retain it as a fashion aid! Stroke patients who have some strength in their affected arm may prefer to hold the stick in that hand, and hold the stick along the line of the affected leg, so that they meet the ground at the same time.

For those who have been unable to avoid contractions of the muscles of the lower leg, a downward pointing foot may be a considerable block to walking. Special footwear, or plastic splints made to fit into the shoes which keep the foot at right angles to the leg, can help them. Calipers for this foot drop are less acceptable, and often restrict full freedom of movement of the leg. For a few patients, however, they may be the only answer.

No chapter on aids for the disabled would be complete without mentioning computers. The most astonishing use of computers in disablement must surely be that by Stephen Hawking, Lucasian

Professor of Mathematics at Cambridge University, and accepted by the whole scientific community as the equal of Einstein as today's leading theoretical physicist. Anyone who might doubt this has only to read his book *A Brief History of Time,* in which he explains his own theories of the origin of the universe and of the meaning of time.

Such work would be difficult enough for a person in robust good health, but Professor Hawking has suffered for more than twenty years from a progressive and incurable nerve disease, amyotrophic lateral sclerosis, that has left him completely paralyzed in all but a few finger movements. His ability to speak was lost several years ago, leaving him only the ability to touch a keyboard fixed to the arm of his electrically-powered wheelchair.

Now, Professor Hawking can converse freely using a voice synthesizer computer, which translates pressure from the keyboard into sounds, which when put together become perfectly understandable speech. Professor Hawking's only complaint, tongue in cheek of course, is that because it was constructed by his American colleagues his speakirig voice now has an American accent!

Professor Hawking's computerized voice is, for the moment, well beyond the financial means of most stroke patients, but it is a sign of things to come. Meanwhile, many stroke patients would benefit by having a simple personal computer to hand.

There are all sorts of ways in which they can be used. First, for simple conversation between a speech-affected patient and his carer.

If understanding of speech has been preserved, and the problem is just one of oral expression, the good hand can be used to type out sentences in response to the conversation around him.

There are computer programs to help patients develop their verbal skills, using question and answer techniques, and computer games using words or pictures are an amusing and absorbing way to improve mental and physical reactions, concentration span, perceptions of space and time, and memory. They can quickly and vastly improve hand-eye co-ordination. Most of all they rekindle the patient's interest in life, provide a variety of intellectual stimuli and challenges, and can greatly boost morale.

Age is no real barrier to starting to use computers: it is a fallacy that the elderly are frightened of new technology. In my experience, most older people rise to the challenge and enjoy the feeling that they can still switch on to the modern world. And if the computer is something that can be shared with the younger generation of visitors, the better the feeling.

Ten years ago, most people would not have considered buying a personal computer. Apart from the cost, which was then prohibitive except for those people in the top tenth of the income range, people looked on computers as beyond their understanding. Now prices have fallen steeply, so that the financial burden is much smaller, and every school-child learns how to work on them at primary school.

The developed nations are fast becoming universally computer literate, and there is no reason why most stroke patients should be left out in the cold. So if families wish to do their best, not just for their stroke victim but in the long term for themselves, they should use what extra money they have and invest in a computer.

# 11 When the Carer Can't Cope

So far, this book has been optimistic. It offers hope for improvement to all stroke victims and their families, and rightly so, because the vast majority of people who survive through the first few days of a stroke recover enough to live a reasonably enjoyable life. Some recover almost completely. The purpose of the previous chapters has been to show how the recovery can be as speedy and as complete as possible.

However, none of this can be achieved without considerable sacrifice by the people closest to the patient, and there are times when that sacrifice can seem, or actually be, too great. It must be admitted that there are stroke victims for whom there is no real recovery, no matter how devoted the family and friends or how much professional time and energy is spent upon them. Even when it is clear that the patient is improving and will be able to stay at home, there are times when the carer needs a break from the arduous task of looking after him.

This chapter, therefore, is devoted to the needs of the carers - spouses, daughters, sons, other family and friends. The great burden of rehabilitation must fall on them: doctors, nurses and other professional therapists, who have only limited time to devote to any one patient, may underestimate or be unable to relieve the mental and physical stress that this can cause.

Realizing that one's spouse has had a stroke is bad enough, but there is sometimes a worse shock to come - on the day that he or she returns home. It is relatively rare for carers to be told beforehand exactly what the management of a stroke victim entails. To have suddenly to care twenty-four hours a day for someone who may have lost mobility, sensation, intellect, ability to communicate and control of bodily functions, and whose character has changed drastically, is very hard to bear.

It is natural for carers to feel bitter and resentful at what has happened: for many spouses the stroke marks the end of all that matters in their marriage, and such bitterness is wholly understandable.

Their difficulty is in expressing their misery without appearing to be disloyal to their partner. If they cannot share their feelings, there is a danger that feelings of guilt, always a destructive emotion, can become overwhelming.

One way to share these feelings is to join a club for relatives of stroke victims: a worry shared is certainly a worry eased in this case. Finding that one is not alone in hating one's life or even one's spouse, and that it is not only common but even normal to react in this way, can assuage the guilt.

Stroke clubs are invaluable in other ways. They can be an introduction to Stroke Volunteers, who can organize off-duty times for carers by taking turns to 'patient sit' . Many also bring the victims together in groups so that they too can compare experiences and help each other to cope. Meanwhile the carers can enjoy some time to themselves. It is not just a chance to be away from the immediate responsibility, but a time to care for themselves and to enjoy their own private lives.

Carers very much need to have this personal life, away from their partners, if they are to do the best for both of them. No partnership can survive for long if one member is only giving and the other only taking. The carer whose life is entirely shaped around a disabled spouse, and who receives nothing in return except total dependency, is in an unacceptable position.

For many carers, this is partly their own fault. They do too much for their stroke-afflicted husbands or wives, so that, instead of being cajoled and stimulated towards helping their own recovery, the invalids sink into a helpless laziness, from which it is difficult to arouse them. Above all, the people around stroke victims must be enthusiastic and be able to transmit that enthusiasm for recovery to them.

When drumming up that enthusiasm has become impossible, either because there is no positive response from the patient or because the stroke has been so severe that recovery seems remote, it is time for the family to take stock. Can they continue, or should they seek some other solution to the patient's long-term care?

Often it is the stress placed on the carer that determines what must happen. Tiredness, irritability, anxiety, appetite loss, sleeplessness, frustration, anger and inability to relax are all signs of stress in carers that strongly suggest that the burden should be shed, at least for a time. If they continue to battle on, the carers themselves may become ill, and this would only serve to double the numbers in the family who need medical care.

In such a position, the family needs help. The decision on future care is usually taken at a case conference, in which doctors, nurses, social workers, health visitors, physiotherapists, and the closest carers all play their part. Either much more help must be arranged in the home, or the patient may have to be placed in a long-stay nursing home or hospital. If this latter course is decided upon, it must be taken with no feelings of guilt. There are times when spouses must let go and leave the caring to the professionals. It is better to do so before the strain has become so great that the rest of the family, and in particular the carer closest to the patient, has been harmed beyond repair.

Nurses will bath and wash the patient. Home helps can take much of the strain from a caring spouse: they do the housework, go shopping, collect prescriptions, and can keep the patient company while the carer is out. Volunteers can bring meals on wheels, others supply laundry services, and still others advise on incontinence and disposal of waste and dressings.

Day hospitals specialize in stroke rehabilitation, training patients to learn again to perform the daily tasks that carers find particularly difficult - such as dressing, shaving, washing, climbing stairs, and using the toilet. Places in day hospitals, which patients take up on one or two days a week, are organized by family doctors or specialists.

Day centers are for groups of more mobile patients. Their aim is to promote social skills with humor and various group activities. The company of others who have been in the same boat and are improving brings some patients out of their shells. Day centers also advise relatives on pensions, social security benefits, other allowances and housing problems. Taking the responsibility for such decisions can remove much of the strain from the carer and can make all the difference to the decision on the future care of the patient.

When it becomes obvious that a spouse has reached her physical and mental limits, the general practitioner may arrange for the hospital to admit the patient for two weeks or so, both to give her a holiday and to subject the patient to more intensive rehabilitation.

This can make a world of difference to the family, especially if it can be arranged at regular intervals - say twice a year. That gives the patient's main carer something concrete to look forward to and to plan for, and may help to avoid or postpone the need for longer hospitalization.

# 12 Final Comments

The big issues are being immobility, instability, incontinence, and intellectual impairment.

The combination is daunting for the rest of the family.

Relatives, must realize the following truths:

- there is no ideal solution
- there is no once and for all solution
- there is no need to feel guilty
- risks cannot be avoided
- the patients must never be forgotten
- family quarrels should be avoided
- money matters.

On the first point, the old person at the center of the crisis is a *person,* not a *problem.* The main concern is to find the least bad outcome for the patient, which may not be the same as finding the solution to the carer's problem.

On the second, a series of gradual and partial improvements in the patient's environment is often better than a radical change which might make matters worse.

On the third, carers who have done their best, perhaps for years, may be made to feel guilty when they finally have to let a spouse or parent go to long-term hospital care. This is especially hard when criticism is led by a relative who lives at a distance and has visited rarely, or by the patient himself. They must push aside any feeling of guilt or failure, and feel happy about the years in which they did provide the care.

As for risks, patients may fall or become ill, or leave the gas on, or even die accidentally. Despite taking every care, a spouse may not be able to prevent such events - and should take them philosophically when they happen.

Not forgetting the patient means being honest and open. Such as *not* telling him he is going for an X-ray or day out when the car is taking him to a long-stay nursing home. Whenever possible the patient should be consulted on all decisions to be made about him.

Watching the situation deteriorate in anguish may be better for a relative than living later with the thought that he removed a loved parent's or spouse's independence before his or her time.

Avoiding arguments within the family during a last illness is essential. In the final days, and afterwards, rows among relatives tend to become permanent estrangements and greatly increase the intensity of the grief. In particular, the one who has done most of the caring should be protected, and other relatives should be supportive rather than jealous or suspicious.

Ten Commandments for all families and carers looking after a disabled member are;

- We shall not fall out.
- We shall not recriminate.
- We shall listen to one another.
- We shall tell one another.
- We shall act together.
- We shall live with the consequences of our decisions.
- We shall give most weight to those who take most responsibility.
- We shall admit when we were wrong.
- We shall give credit where credit is due.
- When all has been said and done we shall feel confident that we acted as best we could in the circumstances in the interests of our patient.

Finally, money. Caring for an elderly invalid at home costs money, just at a time when the subject is not considered 'nice' to bring up. Apart from the extra household costs - such as laundry, fuel bills and travel costs, carers may be put into the position of giving up a job to return home full time. This is often a wrong decision, no matter how correct it appears at the time.

Eventually there is the cost of nursing-home care. Few national health services provide enough beds for the elderly disabled, so that private care can often be the only option. For most individuals the cost of private care is well beyond their reach: either the whole family must chip in or some other source - usually the social security services - must be approached. Families must feel able to talk freely about the financial implications of home care for their patient, and be prepared to share the burden.

"In caring for any elderly invalid, everyone wishes to do what is best: the difficulty is to know what is best, and for whom it is best. If carers take one step at a time, considering each one carefully beforehand, and respecting the wishes of the patient at each step, they will be able to say, at the end: "We did our best because we did what we thought was best". And that, in the end, is all that can be expected of any of us."